SHAPE
Pilates

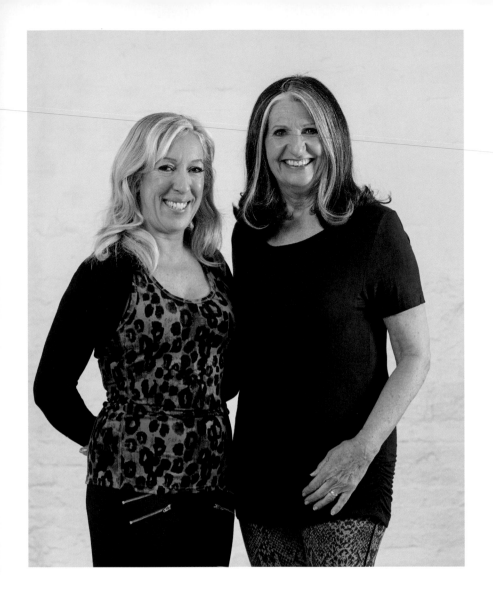

LYNNE ROBINSON is one of the world's most respected Pilates teachers. She is the founder of Body Control Pilates, which is seen as an international benchmark for safe and effective teaching. Her bestselling books include *The Pilates Bible*, *Pilates for Life* and *Pilates for Pregnancy*. She has also produced highly popular DVDs. In demand internationally, she frequently lectures at conferences throughout the world and has taught Pilates in countries as varied as the US, Japan, South Africa, Thailand and Australia.
www.bodycontrolpilates.com

SARAH CLENNELL trained with the Rambert Ballet School and the London School of Contemporary Dance. She trained as a fitness instructor before becoming a teacher trainer for aerobics teachers. She discovered Pilates after a back injury. Qualifying as a Body Control Pilates teacher in 1999, Sarah now teaches on our international teacher training team. In addition to Pilates and aerobics, she has taught Latin and Ballroom Dance, swimming and personal training, giving her 40 years of experience teaching movement!

SHAPE UP
WITH
Pilates

THE ULTIMATE GUIDE
TO **SCULPTING,**
STRENGTHENING
& STREAMLINING
YOUR BODY

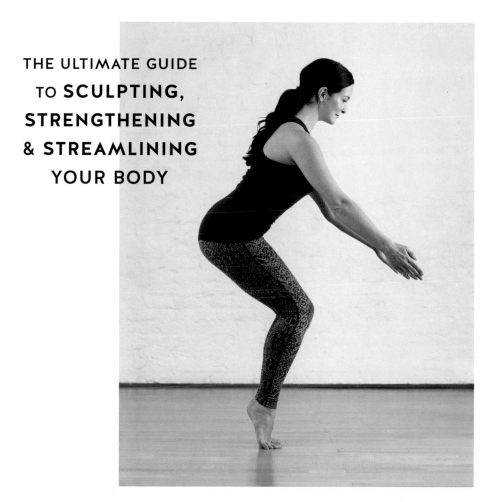

LYNNE ROBINSON

PILATES CONSULTANT: SARAH CLENNELL
NUTRITION EXPERT: HELEN FORD BA HONS, DIP ION, MBANT, CNHC

Contents

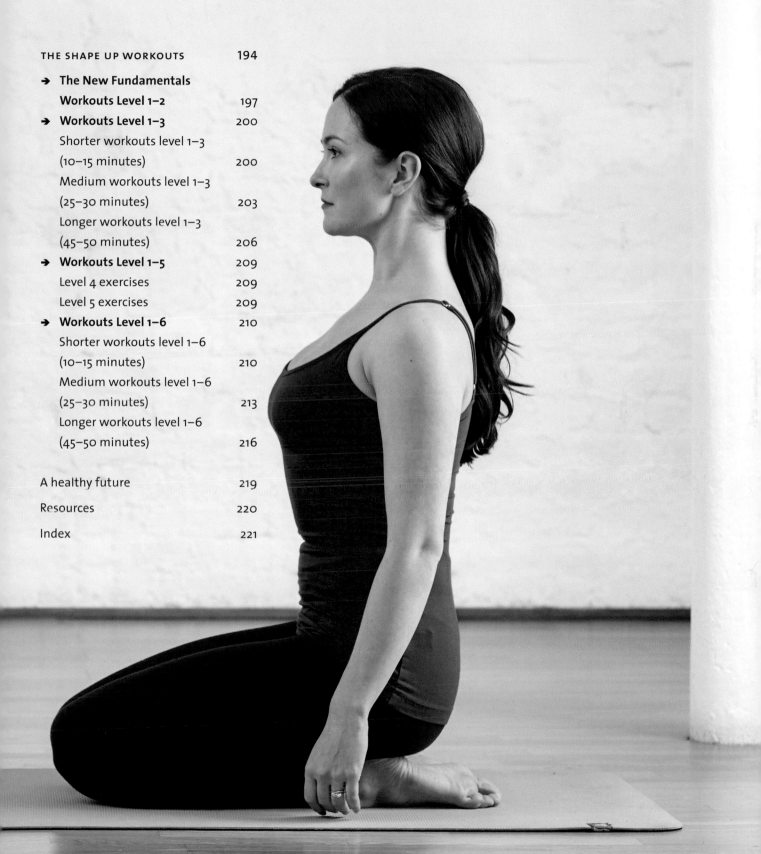

Introduction

Everyone deserves to be happy with their body, regardless of its size and shape, and free from the pressure of friends, family, social media and fashion. We are who we are, unique and wondrously different.

However, we also owe it to ourselves and our families – even to society – to be healthy and in the best shape we can be; to be supple, strong and fit to enjoy life. We have written this book to empower you to achieve not just the body of your dreams but optimal health. This was Joseph Pilates' goal – he believed his method could "wake" us up and "return us to life".

"Physical fitness is the first requisite of happiness. Our interpretation of physical fitness is the attainment and maintenance of a uniformly developed body with a sound mind fully capable of naturally, easily and satisfactorily performing our many and varied daily tasks with spontaneous zest and pleasure."

JOSEPH PILATES, *RETURN TO LIFE THROUGH CONTROLOGY*

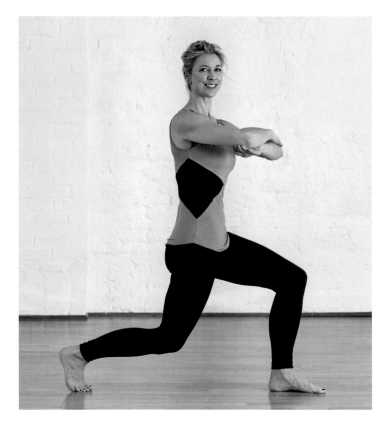

The transformation will not happen overnight and it cannot be bought – it has to be earned through regular practice and a determination to live more healthily. But if you can give us three months, we can help you not only sculpt your body, but achieve optimum wellness.

You will feel the benefits of this exciting new exercise programme within the first few weeks. You'll look taller and fitter, and others will notice the change. Within three months you will look and feel like a new person. And the results will last!

Do you have a dream body in mind? You are not alone. There has always been huge pressure on women to look "attractive" – our great-great-grandmothers laced themselves into corsets so tight they could hardly breathe! But the pressure to look good 24/7 has never been greater than now, when our images are out there on social media and there is nowhere to hide.

Thank heavens then for the growing body positivity movement celebrating diversity. In this book, our models are different shapes and sizes but they have one thing in common. They all exercise regularly and are in great shape.

So take a moment to think about what you really want. Is that a six-pack or simply a flatter tummy? Arms like a boxer or subtly sculpted arms? Perhaps you want to streamline your silhouette, but retain its natural curves.

It's your body and your choice. We want to celebrate your natural shape while helping you refine and define it. The Shape Up programme will help you reveal the shape you want to be.

WHO IS THIS BOOK FOR?

You! Whether you are new to Pilates or a veteran, here is a book bursting with valuable tips and exciting new exercises. This is Body Control Pilates at its most creative, innovative and authoritative. Clear teaching points have made our books bestsellers, and this one is no exception. We'll share our years of experience teaching Pilates as if we were right there by your side.

Step-by-step, day-by-day, week-by-week, we will guide you. The workout plan is simple to follow, with Pilates sessions that slot easily into your weekly routine. The dietary advice is equally straightforward and achievable, and the lifestyle tips life-changing, even life-saving!

We will introduce you to the New Fundamentals of Body Control Pilates, the essential exercises for top-to-toe mind and body conditioning, and ways to adapt them to increase their challenge and toning power. We appreciate that you may decide to tone some parts of your body more than others, so there are special sections on the abdominals, waist, arms and shoulders, buttocks, thighs and calves, and the back... no body part escapes our attention in this nose-to-tail approach! We have had a huge amount of fun exploring new ways to help you tone up.

Then you take control, deciding how often, when and for how long to do the workouts. You can choose

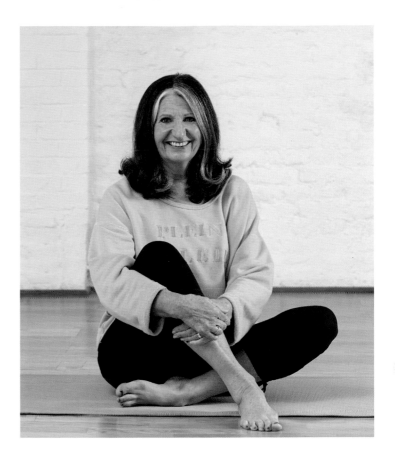

"Lynne is the only woman on earth who has ever got my stomach looking anywhere near flat, so I think of her as something of a miracle worker."
KATE REW, AUTHOR AND JOURNALIST

short daily workouts, slightly longer workouts five days a week, or perhaps you'd prefer three 45-minute weekly sessions. You just have to do 150 minutes (2½ hours) of Pilates each week. Combined with cardiovascular activities and a healthy diet, this is the perfect recipe for health.

We don't make unrealistic promises – we are looking for lasting changes that set you up to stay in shape for life. No more yo-yo dieting, no more punishing workouts. Instead, you'll understand your body and work with it in a holistic, achievable and sustainable way.

All you need to achieve the body of your dreams is 12 weeks and the commitment to follow the plan.

"In 10 sessions you'll feel the difference, in 20 you'll see the difference, in 30 you'll have a whole new body."

JOSEPH PILATES, *RETURN TO LIFE THROUGH CONTROLOGY*

WHAT MAKES THIS SHAPE UP PROGRAMME DIFFERENT?

Your Pilates sessions will never be the same again! This programme is packed with new exercises hand-picked for their power to tone muscle. We've added a cardio element by applying Pilates principles to popular gym exercises like Lunges and Squats. And to achieve maximum results in minimum time, we've added more challenge to old Pilates favourites by combining movements and sequencing exercises. For example, you can do Table Top from the New Fundamentals as a simple exercise (see page 74), or add extra challenge and toning power by combining it with a Salute and Knee bend (see page 77) or even a Flies variation with weights (see page 145).

Some of the new combinations will also be very welcome to those of you who are hard pressed for time. For example, by combining a Ribcage Closure with Knee Rolls (page 73), you are gently mobilizing your hips and shoulders in one go. Great for the warm up phase of your workouts.

We've also sequenced exercises, following one movement immediately with another to target more muscles per exercise. For example, the sequence of Arm Weight exercises on pages 151–155 targets the biceps, triceps, shoulder and chest muscles. Opt to squeeze a pillow between your knees as you practise and you'll be working your inner thighs too!

Building on the basics in the New Fundamentals, we add challenge after challenge by reducing the base of support – for example Cat (page 95) becomes One-armed Cat (page 96), Bridge (see page 158) becomes Pretzel Bridge (page 160), and Wall Push Ups (page 146) become One Arm Wall Push Ups (page 147).

We've added extra load with hand weights and resistance with stretch bands. Then there are lots of exciting new exercises, such as Back Bridge (see page 162), which is wonderful for toning your buttocks, core and arms. Each exercise has a level of difficulty (1–6) so you can work comfortably at your own pace, making layer upon layer of fun challenges.

A BALANCED HEALTHY LIFE

We are not just concerned with shape – we want you to feel as amazing as you look, and achieve optimum health and fitness. Joseph Pilates understood this, writing not just about his exercise method "Contrology" in his books *Your Health* and *Return to Life through Contrology*, but also about the multiple benefits of a healthy lifestyle

Joseph Pilates wrote these books in 1934 and 1945 respectively. Reading them now, you realize how much sound lifestyle advice they contain, which is now being reinforced by research. It's taken decades for the world to catch up.

Joe wasn't perfect. He smoked cigars and drank quite heavily, but to reach 79 years of age with a physique that would be the envy of a 40-year-old, he must have been doing something right. So to honour his legacy, maximize your shaping up and ensure optimum wellness, in addition to the Shape Up exercise programme, you'll find advice on healthy eating (see pages 28–33), the link between stress, health and weight gain, and the importance of sleep, fresh air, sunlight and darkness, with practical tips on bringing these essentials into your life.

We hope that by doing regular Pilates you will be more in tune with your body and understand your

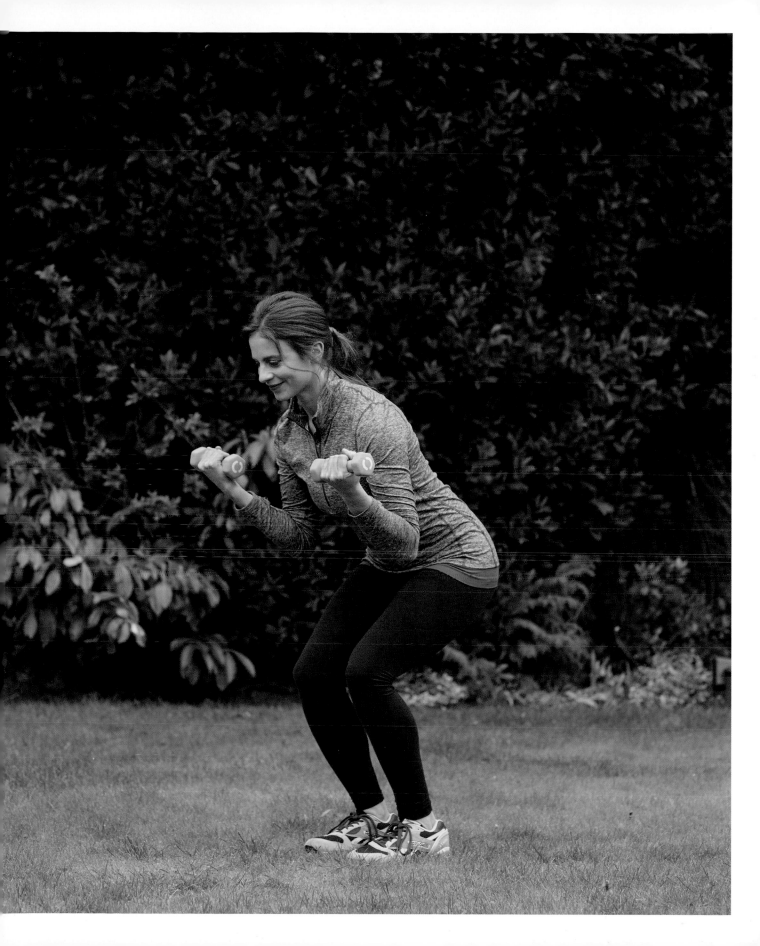

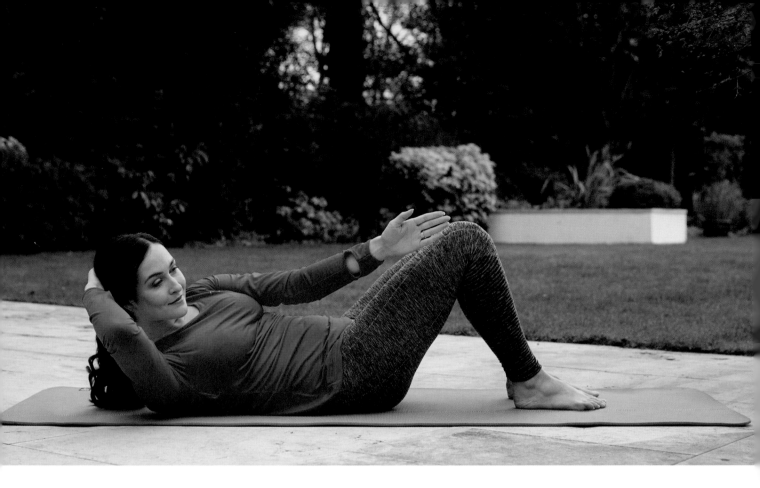

natural rhythms and needs. I have found, and my clients have also reported, that the heightened mind–body connection Pilates gives can help you make the right lifestyle choices. You recognize signs of tiredness, which helps you decide when you need sleep and for how long. You'll notice when you are getting stressed and know what to do to help control it. Being more body-aware can also help you make the right food choices.

It's not foolproof – there will be times when you feel stressed, tired and hungry and your body craves sweet, salty, fatty things – but I have a motto that has served me well over time: "Eat first what you should, and then what you would". If I follow this rule, I find my body feels nourished and I have fewer unhealthy cravings.

There is nothing new in the concept of regular exercise and a balanced diet for health. Hippocrates of Greece (460–370 BCE) was the first "recorded" physician to provide a written exercise prescription for a patient.

While in 600 BCE, the Indian physician Sushruta was concerned that individuals who consumed too much food, slept too long and remained sedentary while pampering their bellies would become corpulent, a condition he associated with a variety of diseases, and for which he prescribed exercise, stating that "diseases fly from the presence of a person habituated to regular physical exercise".

More recently, in 2007, the American College of Sports Medicine, with endorsement from the American Medical Association and the Office of the Surgeon General, launched a global initiative to mobilize physicians and healthcare professionals to promote exercise in their practice. Out of this initiative came the term Exercise Is Medicine and the recommendation that healthy adults perform 150 minutes of moderate dynamic exercise each week. This advice still stands across the globe.

SHAPE UP AND LOSE WEIGHT OR JUST SHAPE UP?

Before we begin the Shape Up programme we should be clear about our objectives. You will have read often that, in order to shape up and lose weight, you need to exercise more and eat less. But emerging research suggests that it's far more complicated than the simple equation of burning more calories than we consume. Remember too that you can be slim and yet out of shape and very unfit, or in shape and fit but register as overweight on a chart. The relationship between weight and weight loss is complex. We will be exploring this in depth later in the book.

For now, suffice to say that by following this programme, we want to make your body more efficient at burning the food you consume by improving your metabolic rate. To do this, you need to create lean body mass – the muscle mass beneath your body fat that burns calories day in, day out, even when you're resting. Muscle requires more blood and oxygen than fat, increasing the energy the body has to expend to maintain it.

For long-term success, you need the right muscle mass to maintain this high metabolic rate. If you starve yourself you may lose body fat and weigh less on the scales, but without a strength-training routine like Pilates you will also lose the muscle resources needed to keep your metabolic rate high. In fact, your metabolic rate may slow, then you may not be able to maintain the weight loss because every time you eat a few extra calories, you pile the pounds back on.

You may not burn quite as many calories doing a Pilates session as running, but the many standing exercises in this book, especially the new Lunges and Squats, will help. With the increased repetitions you'll also build muscle tissue from top to toe, enabling you to burn calories 24/7 even after finishing a workout.

BENEFITS OF REGULAR PILATES AS REPORTED BY OUR CLIENTS

- Improved body awareness.
- Better posture.
- Increased flexibility and strength in the spine.
- Improved joint mobility, resulting in fewer joint aches and pains.
- Better balance and coordination.
- More efficient breathing and all the health and beauty benefits that brings.
- Improved bone strength.
- Increased stamina and energy.
- Stronger muscles, in particular the gluteals, quadriceps, hamstrings, calves, upper arm muscles, back, and of course the abdominal muscles and pelvic floor.
- More streamlined outline, in particular a defined waistline.
- Healthier, less painful feet.
- Improved sleep patterns.
- Increased self-esteem and confidence.
- Less stress and better mental health.
- Increased feeling of health and wellbeing.

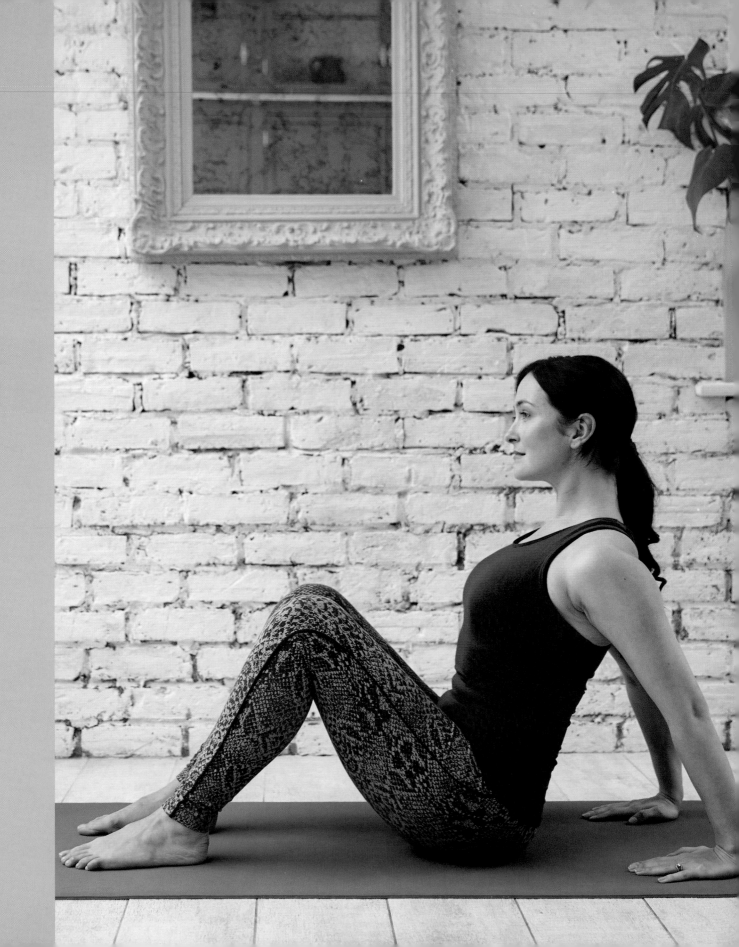

SHAPE UP
Lifestyle

A good night's sleep

*"... proper diet and sufficient sleep must supplement our exercise
in our quest for physical fitness... [the person] who uses intelligence
with respect to diet, sleeping habits and who exercises properly,
is beyond any question of doubt taking the very best preventative
medicines provided so freely and abundantly by nature."*

JOSEPH PILATES, *RETURN TO LIFE THROUGH CONTROLOGY*

Joseph Pilates extolled the virtues of a good night's sleep for good health – though, he would have us all sleeping in a deep V-shaped bed! He felt that among the most important requirements for a good night's sleep are quiet, darkness, fresh air and mental calm.

A good night's sleep may also play a role in weight management. Doctors have known for some time that many hormones are affected by how well we sleep, but production of leptin and ghrelin, hormones that work together to control feelings of hunger and satiety, may be particularly influential. Ghrelin, produced in the gastrointestinal tract, stimulates our appetite, while leptin, produced in fat cells, sends signals to the brain to indicate when we are full. If you fail to get enough sleep, leptin levels can drop, meaning you may still feel hungry despite having eaten sufficient quantities of food. At the same time, lack of sleep causes ghrelin levels in the body to rise, stimulating the appetite.

Quality of sleep counts, too. A decreased amount of time spent in restorative deep or slow-wave sleep has been associated with significantly reduced levels of growth hormone, a protein that helps the adult body to regulate proportions of fat and muscle.

Overall health suffers from lack of sleep. When we sleep, fluids are driven through the brain, flushing out toxins, and similar processes take place throughout the body. If we don't get enough sleep, these natural processes are disrupted, and our minds and bodies suffer. For wellbeing, we need to respect our circadian rhythm, the inner biological clock that helps to regulate our body systems (see page 18).

How much sleep do you need? Researchers agree that the optimum amount varies for each of us. Some people can thrive on six hours a night, while others need eight or even nine. Only you can tell whether you are getting enough.

TIPS FOR BETTER SLEEP

- Establish a bedtime routine and a regular bedtime – adults need this just as much as children.

- Set a regular time to wake up, and avoid going to bed later and waking later at weekends. This can upset your body clock in a similar way to jet lag.

- Engage in relaxing activities before bed, such as reading, listening to music or doing a few gentle Pilates exercises (see page 16).

- Avoid thrillers, anything too exciting on TV or cardiovascular activities that get the heart racing for about three hours before bedtime.

- Steer clear of caffeine also in the evening (note that green tea and white tea contain caffeine).

- Have a proper meal in the evening (not too late) so that that you do not go to bed hungry. But don't snack before bedtime. It may sit heavy on your stomach.

- Take a power nap mid-afternoon if you find it beneficial, but not if you have trouble sleeping at night.

- Be aware that alcohol disturbs your sleep cycle. It sedates the cortex of the brain, but sedation is not sleep. It can also suppress REM, deep dream sleep.

- Make your bedroom temperature conducive to sleep: a cool 18°C (64.4°F) helps bring your body temperature down, encouraging sleep.

- Take a hot bath to bring blood to the surface of your skin. The dilated blood vessels radiate out your inner core heat, which drops your body temperature.

- Sleep in the dark to encourage the release of melatonin, the hormone that regulates the onset of the sleep cycle.

- Ban "blue-light" technology – screens on phones, laptops, tablets and digital clocks – from about 30 minutes before retiring and from the bedroom. Blue light can block the release of melatonin so your brain doesn't recognize evening as bedtime.

- Consider removing all clocks from view if you find yourself checking the time in the night.

- Get enough sunlight during the day to enhance your circadian rhythm (see page 18).

- Make sure your mattress and pillow are comfortable. Try a selection to find the best for you – while a firmer mattress may be better for your back, it can be hard on the joints.

- Consider sleeping on your left side, suggested in studies to help flush toxins from the brain so that you wake feeling more refreshed.

- Write a list if your mind cannot switch off. Committing tasks to paper can help organize thoughts and stop you worrying. Write the list in another room, finishing with happy thoughts of positive things that happened that day or week. Leave the list in the other room before going to bed.

- Get up if you cannot drop off to sleep after about 30 minutes. Read an unexciting book (in another room so the bedroom is reserved for sleep), go for a gentle stroll or try a few Pilates moves. I have been told my voice can be soporific, so try listening to my chill-out exercises online at Body Control Pilates Central (www.bodycontrolpilatescentral.vhx.tv).

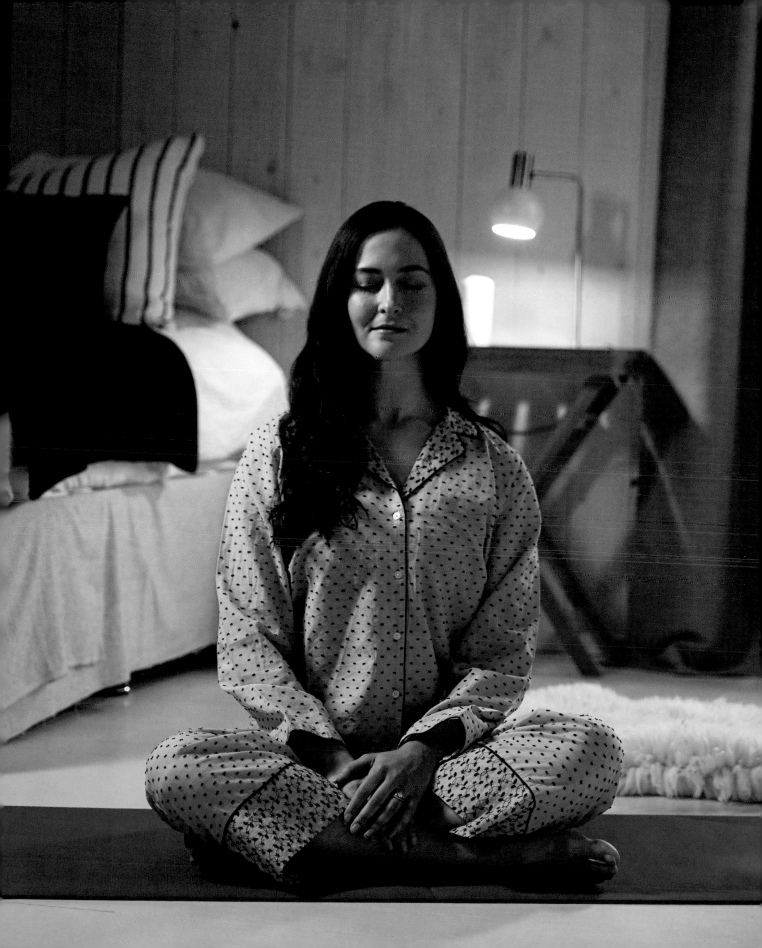

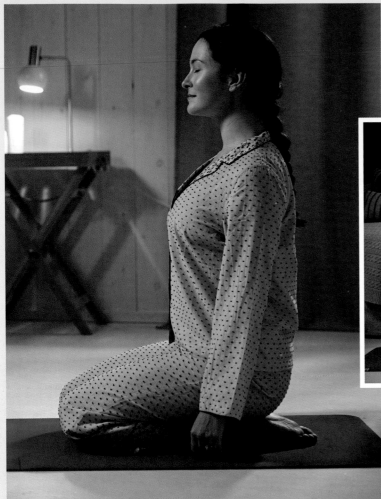

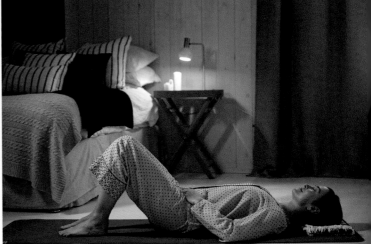

PILATES EXERCISES FOR GOOD SLEEP

- Relaxation Position (page 48)
- Chin Tucks and Neck Rolls (page 52)
- Knee Rolls (page 73)
- Shoulder Drops (page 78)
- Leg Slides (page 68)
- Spine Curls (page 90)
- Cat (page 95)
- Lizard (page 178)
- Rest Position (page 108)
- Cobra Prep with Neck Turn (page 175)
- Hip Rolls with Ribcage Closure (page 103)
- Arm Openings (page 100)
- Side Reach (page 104)
- Roll Downs (page 110)

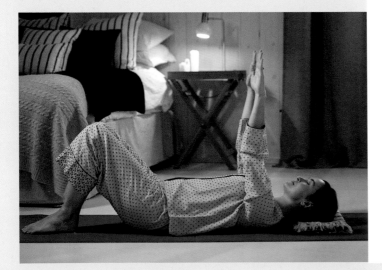

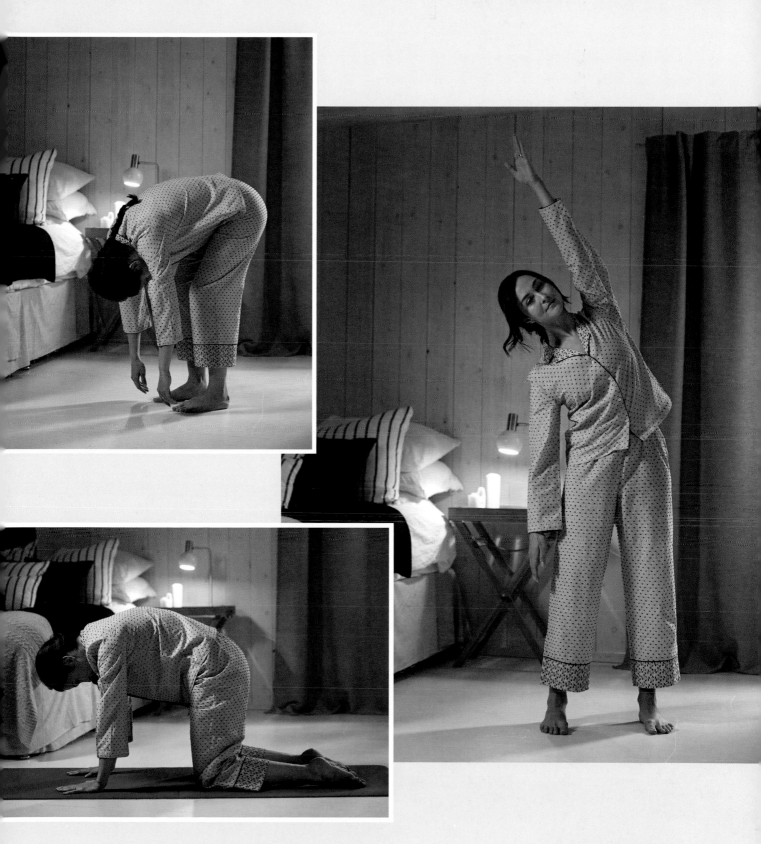

Fresh air, sunlight & darkness

*"By all means never fail to get all the sunshine
and fresh air that you can."*

JOSEPH PILATES, *RETURN TO LIFE THROUGH CONTROLOGY*

In our archives are lots of photographs of Joseph Pilates working out – a great many show him outdoors exercising in his swimming trunks. He wanted to show off his fine, muscled physique, but he also understood the benefits of fresh air and sunshine.

As a child Joe suffered with rickets, the bone disorder caused by, among other factors, lack of vitamin D (sunlight triggers the body to manufacture this vitamin). Joe also sported a good suntan in the summer months. We are more apprehensive about sun damage these days because of links to skin cancer, but our bodies do need some sunlight to thrive.

In her 2019 book *Chasing the Sun*, journalist Linda Geddes explains how sunlight shapes our bodies and minds. She argues that because modern daytimes are too dark and nights too bright, we have lost touch with our natural circadian rhythm, the inner biological clock that regulates our organs.

Before the invention of gaslight and then electricity, our predecessors rose with the dawn and went to bed at nightfall (candles were costly). These days we are rarely in the dark for long and many of us spend too little time outside in sunlight. Geddes explains that this has a negative effect on our wellbeing and argues that lack of sunlight has contributed to, among other things, short-sightedness among East Asian children and the higher incidence of the autoimmune disease multiple sclerosis in the population of countries further from the equator. Shift workers also have increased health risks, including mental health problems, obesity, heart disease and cancer.

It's relatively simple to adapt the home and workplace to fit our circadian rhythm with natural daylight bulbs and by turning lights down in the evening. But it's more important to spend as much time as you can outdoors. The rise of forest schools where children learn outdoors in all weathers and temperatures, rain or shine, is something we can learn from, like the Japanese practice of *shinrin-yoku*, spending time in the forest to promote health. It originated in the 1980s as a national health programme and 2.5 million people in Japan are said to practise "forest bathing" every year.

There is proof of the benefits to mental health of being in nature. Joint research from the University of Madrid and the Norwegian University of Life Sciences (2007) revealed that simply seeing a natural landscape has the potential to speed recovery from mental fatigue and stress, while in the UK, University of Exeter studies showed that putting vegetation in an urban environment lessened perceived levels of anxiety, depression and stress among city occupants.

Try to spend at least two hours a week outdoors in nature (woods, parks or the countryside). This is the minimum time needed to be beneficial for your health and psychological wellbeing, lowering stress levels and blood pressure, according to research from the University of Exeter (2019 *Scientific Reports*).

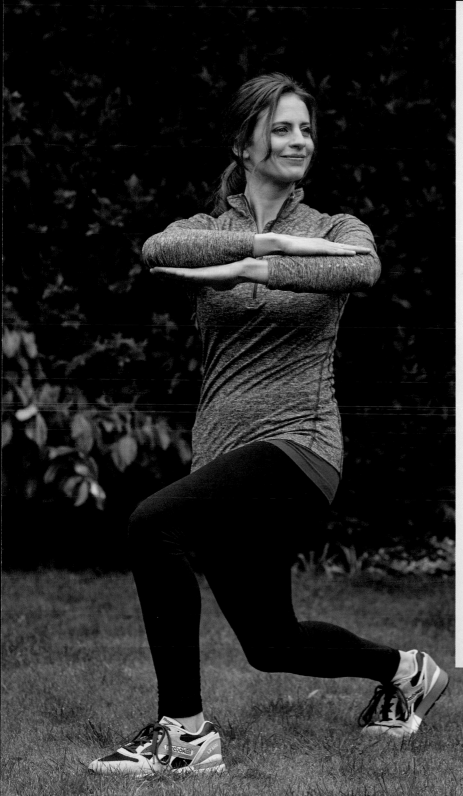

TIPS FOR EXERCISING OUTSIDE

- Pick outdoor cardio activities. A brisk walk through the woods is preferable to a brisk walk on a treadmill, cycling outdoors is better than a stationary bike, and lawn tennis beats squash.

- Do not allow the weather to put you off being outside. The Norwegians have a saying "There is no such thing as bad weather, only wrong clothing!"

- Wrap up in layers that allow you to move freely, discarding or adding more as necessary (we aren't all as hardy as Joe).

- In summer, pick a shady spot; don't exercise in full sun or the heat of the day, even wearing sunscreen. Exercising in the early morning or later afternoon minimizes the risk of sun damage. Drink plenty of water.

- In cooler months, some gentle sunshine is welcome for overall health and our bones – try to get 10 minutes daily.

- Look for flat ground to lay your Pilates mat (you may need two) so you can find your neutral pelvis and spine.

- Opt for standing Pilates exercises if you cannot find enough flat ground for a mat.

- If wearing shoes for outdoor Pilates, choose flexible soles so you can roll through your feet.

STANDING OUTDOOR MINI WORKOUT

- The Leg Shaper (page 156)
- Standing Pilates Stance Arm Circles (page 84)
- Standing Side Reach (page 104)
- Pilates Squat with Bicep Curls (page 169)
- Waist Twists in Static Standing Lunge (page 98)
- Dynamic Lunges with Double Floating Arms (page 172)
- Roll Downs into Standing Back Bend with Arm Circles (page 185)

See also the suggested exercises for before and after a walk or run in the Cardiovascular section on page 186.

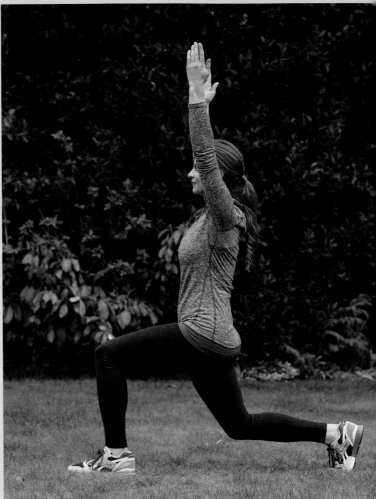

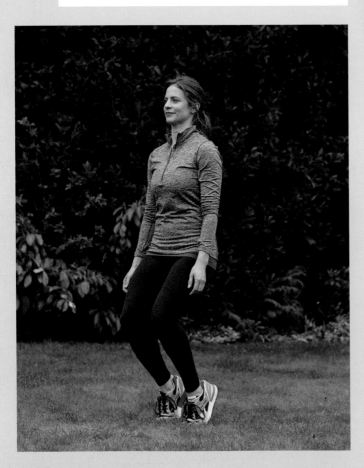

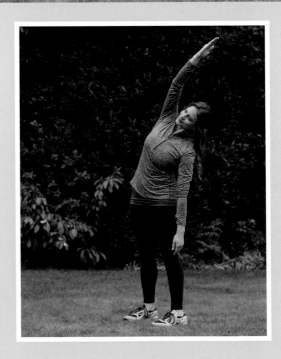

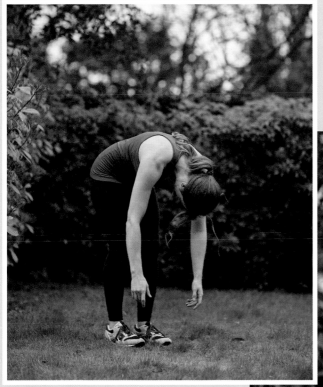

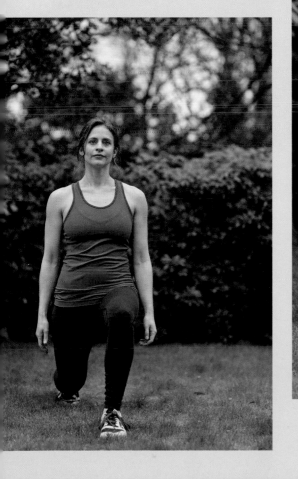

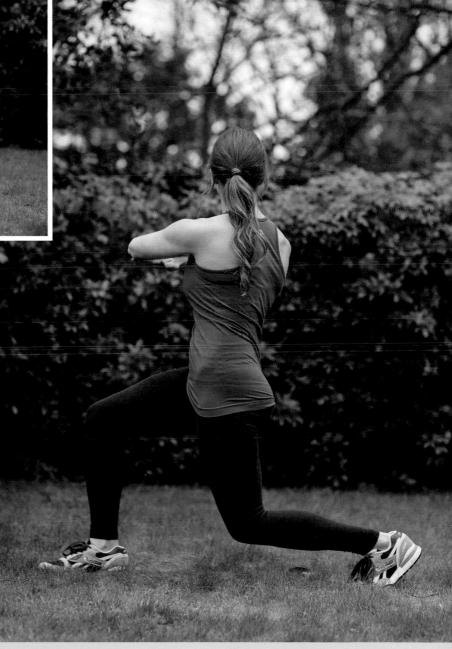

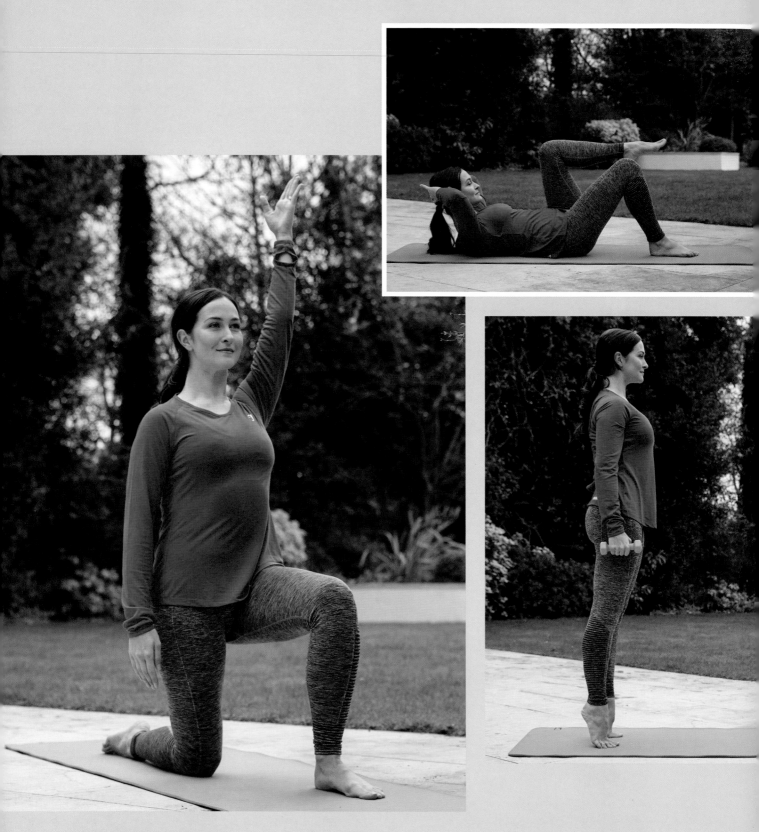

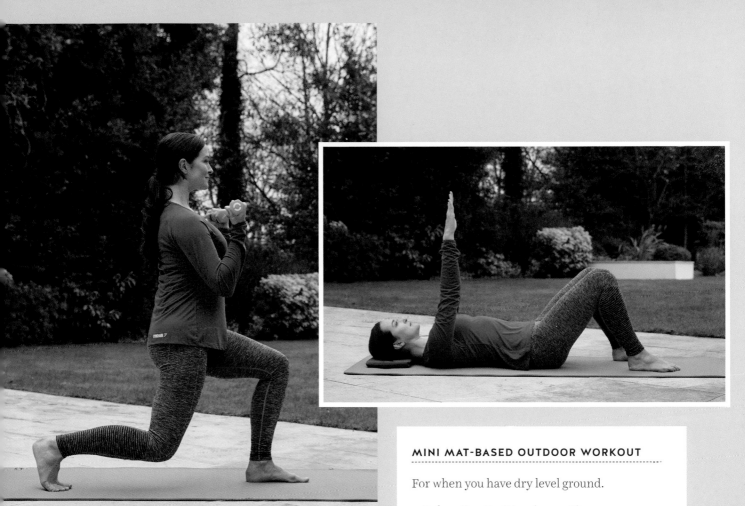

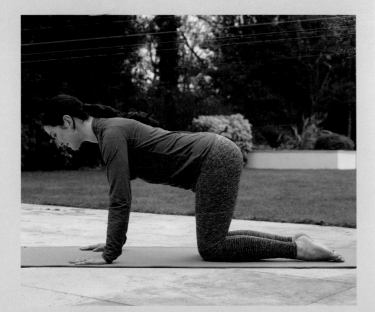

MINI MAT-BASED OUTDOOR WORKOUT

For when you have dry level ground.

- Relaxation Position (page 48)
- Chin Tucks and Neck Rolls (page 52)
- Knee Rolls with Ribcage Closure (page 73)
- Curl Ups with Single Knee Fold (page 93)
- Oblique Curl Ups with Reach (page 117)
- Butterflies (page 101)
- Diamond Press Salute (page 107)
- Box Push Ups (page 150)
- High Kneeling Lunge Side Reach (page 105)
- Dynamic Lunges with Biceps Curls
  (page 173)
- Roll Downs with Weights (page 112)

Stress, health & weight management

"A body free from nervous tension and fatigue is the ideal shelter provided by nature for housing a well-balanced mind, fully capable of successfully meeting all the complex problems of modern living."

JOSEPH PILATES, *RETURN TO LIFE THROUGH CONTROLOGY*

The World Health Organization (WHO) calls stress "the health epidemic of the 21st century". But we need to look deeper to understand how stress can make us put on weight and how exercise – in particular, Pilates – can help relieve the effects of stress.

Modern lifestyles expose us to daily stressors our bodies aren't designed to put up with long term. We evolved to survive periods of short-term acute stress. Ongoing chronic stress puts more pressure on the adrenal glands (stress glands) and triggers the production of adrenaline, the fight or flight hormone, and cortisol, a fat-storing hormone produced in response to too much stress and fluctuating blood-sugar levels.

Stress itself is not bad. As a response to potential danger it is a basic survival tool. When our ancestors faced their woolly mammoths or sabre-toothed tigers, their bodies responded by preparing to fight or flee. Part of the brain, the hypothalamus, is activated, the hormone adrenocorticotrophic is released from the pituitary, which acts on the adrenals to produce stress hormones. Sugars are released into the blood so we can run faster or fight harder. At the same time muscle and liver cells become resistant to the hormone insulin, so the sugars remain in the bloodstream. The heart beats faster, blood pressure rises and any non-essential bodily functions switch off (we may be sick to save energy on digestion or we may need the bathroom). Fighting – or running away from – the mammoth or tiger dissipates the stress reactions.

The type of stress we meet most often now has changed. While we might occasionally be subjected to an event where the fight or flight response would save our lives, for the most part we face long-term stress that isn't relieved by fighting or running away. That might be from working long hours, financial or marital problems, worry about the kids, or technology that makes it hard to leave the office behind.

Chronic stress weakens the immune system, accelerates ageing and can cause metabolic changes that lead to weight gain. If you are on the go all day, every day, you might think the busy activity would help you lose weight. Instead, chronic stress interferes with your hunger and satiety (feeling full) messengers, making you crave certain foods. And, sadly, it is not broccoli we crave when stressed, but comfort foods high in sugar and fat.

Stress encourages the body to store extra calories as fat, in the belief that being stressed indicates hard times ahead, perhaps famine. And of course, it stores the fat in all the familiar places: midriff, abdomen, upper thighs, hips and buttocks. If this state of chronic stress continues, you leave yourself open to increased risk of obesity, type 2 diabetes, high blood pressure, insomnia, depression, anxiety and heart disease. Short-term inflammation, the result of your immune system firing up to help you recover quickly (in case that sabre-toothed tiger got the better of you), can go on to become chronic inflammation, linked to DNA damage.

TIPS FOR STRESS RELIEF

- Do just 10 minutes a day of mindfulness meditation or mindful exercise like Pilates, yoga or tai chi.

- Learn when to say no – learn to delegate and when you do have a particular burden, try sharing it with others.

- Boost your self-esteem, especially if you find yourself in a negative spiral of self-doubt. Remind yourself of times you successfully tackled problems and surround yourself with positive people who help and reassure you.

- Go to sleep on happy thoughts, listing all the wonderful things that happened today and that you plan to do tomorrow.

- Adopt healthy-eating patterns, eating mindfully and at regular intervals, and choosing foods that stabilize your blood-sugar levels (see page 30). But be careful not to get stressed trying to follow too strict a diet.

- Build magnesium into your diet. 400mg may relax the body and help symptoms of depression. Good food sources include oats, bananas and kidney beans.

- Put your phone down, especially when out with friends and during meals. You might consider a digital curfew between 9pm and 8am.

- Schedule some spa time to relax and be pampered.

- When one part of life, say work, is making you feel stressed, put more energy into areas still under your control, such as gardening, decorating or Pilates.

- Put time and effort into connecting with family and friends – relationships with the people we love lie at the very heart of our happiness.

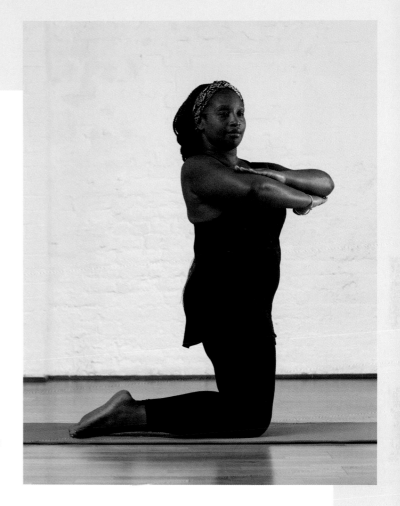

- Sample how good it feels to give by donating time to your favourite charity.

- Try meditation or mindfulness classes (or an app or book). The health benefits are almost too numerous to mention, including lowering blood pressure, heart rate and levels of cortisol and other stress hormones. It also helps you focus on your movements during Pilates practice.

- Laugh more, possibly the ultimate remedy for stress. If you cannot remember your last fall-off-the-chair belly laugh it's time to plan some serious fun.

Mindful wellbeing through exercise

"It is the spirit itself which shapes the body."

JOSEPH PILATES, *RETURN TO LIFE THROUGH CONTROLOGY*

One day a year at a spa can only do so much destressing – we need a more permanent solution to avoid stress-related illness and control our weight. Exercise, in any form, is a very useful way of reducing stress levels. By stimulating the reward centre of the brain, exercise produces endorphins, the feel-good hormones. It also leads to an increase in stress-reducing serotonin and norepinephrine, which make us feel happier.

What's more, when we challenge ourselves with workouts, the mind and body can practise responding to stress, making us better able to cope with difficult situations in other areas of life. This is why we have included more challenging options in the Shape Up programme and recommend adding aerobic exercise to your weekly routine.

Pilates regulars have always told us they feel calm, relaxed and happier after sessions. We always assumed this was a combination of post-exercise feel-good hormones and the calming breathing techniques we teach. But 2016 research from the University of Pittsburgh, in the USA, gave fresh insight into why Pilates (and other mind–body practices) leave us feeling free from stress.

The Pittsburgh research provided evidence for the neural basis of the mind–body connection, discovering a circuit that directly links the cerebral cortex part of the brain to the inner part of the adrenal gland that triggers the adrenal surge when we are faced with danger. It seems that this very same brain network is also associated with the motor cortex controlling movement. The research may explain why meditation and exercises like yoga and Pilates can help modulate the body's responses to physical, mental and emotional stress.

Mindfulness is increasingly recognized as having huge benefits for health. But there appears to be a profound link between mindfulness and weight management. In a 2018 University of Warwick, in the UK study, participants of an obesity programme who also took mindfulness sessions lost more weight over six months than those who simply followed the programme.

What exactly is mindfulness? It can be described as a mind–body practice in which you learn enhanced awareness: of your current state of mind, your body and your environment. This can be achieved through sitting meditation, but also through mindful exercise such as Pilates, yoga and tai chi.

Pilates is a mind–body technique that incorporates mindfulness with every movement. You have to be totally in the moment, aware of your breath, your posture and your movements. For anyone who finds meditation difficult – and I count myself within this group – Pilates offers a great alternative approach. We might call it meditation through movement.

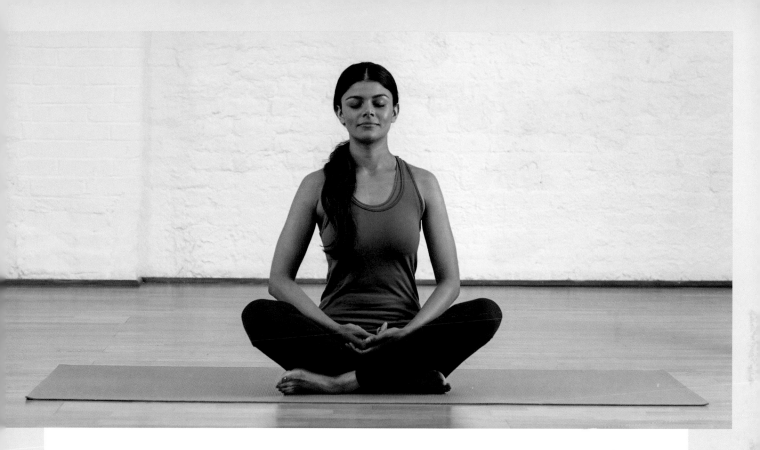

SIMPLE MEDITATION

Find a quiet place where you will not be disturbed. The room should be warm, softly lit and well ventilated. Consider recording the instructions so you can relax while following them.

1   Sit comfortably on a chair, with both feet on the floor, or sit with crossed legs on a mat. Use cushions for support and to keep your spine upright or rest your back against a wall. Or try the meditation lying down. I like to have a large pillow under my knees.

2   Close your eyes and relax the muscles of your jaw and face. Allow your tongue to widen at its base.

3   Bring your awareness to the gentle ebb and flow of your breath. Feel your abdomen expand as you inhale. Gently allow the breath to flow out through your mouth.

4   Make your exhalation twice as long as your inhalation. Empty your lungs, then feel new breath filling your lungs. Breathe slowly, counting as you inhale and exhale.

4   One by one, empty your mind of worries accumulated during the day until you can focus on a single positive thought, image or affirmation.

5   If you like, repeat the ancient Sanskrit mantra "OM" as one long, drawn-out sound. Feel it reverberate through you.

6   When ready, gradually become aware of your surroundings. Tune in first to the sounds and scents, then open your eyes.

7   Start to move your body gradually, then, if lying, roll onto your side and rest a moment before slowly standing up or, if seated, stand up slowly and mindfully.

Food for health

Regular mindful exercise helps unite mind and body in such a way that you start to become aware of your natural rhythms, including becoming more attuned to when and how often you need to eat and which foods are good for you.

It's important to enjoy food. The eating experience in its entirety should satisfy mind, body and soul, and be seen as a pleasure – not just fuel to get you from A to B. Mindful eating is the first step. You can't appreciate a meal when distracted, and eating in front of a screen or while working is not conducive to a healthy digestive system. It's also easy to overeat when you're not focused on what you're putting in your mouth. We should aim instead for the prolonged and sociable mealtimes with the whole family that are a feature of so many Mediterranean countries.

The health of your gut can influence your weight as well as overall health. Research into the gut microbiome – the combination of good and bad bacteria in the intestines – shows it can be altered by diet and stress levels. A study* took two groups of mice of the same weight, and fed one a diet to make them obese and the other a diet to make them skinny. The gut microbiome from the obese mice was then put into the skinny mice. The skinny mice continued their skinny diet but became obese. This is exciting because it suggests that by nurturing the gut with good food and stress-relieving mindful eating we can positively influence our health and weight.

Fasting is a trend that may support weight loss and improve blood sugar, brain function and longevity. Our favourite is 16/8 intermittent fasting, which involves eating during an eight-hour window and fasting for the remaining 16 hours. This seems more manageable than plans such as the 5/2 day fast, where binge eating can be common.

It's thought that during fast periods insulin sensitivity improves, preventing the spikes and dips experienced by so many people. Between meals, as long as we don't snack, our insulin levels go down and fat cells release stored sugar to be used as energy. We lose weight if we let our insulin levels go down far enough for long enough that we burn off fat. The resulting overall reduction in calorie intake (if you don't overeat during the eating window) is also helpful. As with any new eating plan, do seek advice from your medical practitioner before starting, especially if you have a health condition.

* P Lu, C P Sodhi, Y Yamaguchi, H Jia, T Prindle, W B Fulton, A Vikram, K J Bibby, M J Morowitz, D J Hackam, "Intestinal epithelial Toll-like receptor 4 prevents metabolic syndrome by regulating interactions between microbes and intestinal epithelial cells in mice", *Mucosal Immunology*, 2018; DOI: 10.1038/mi.2017.114

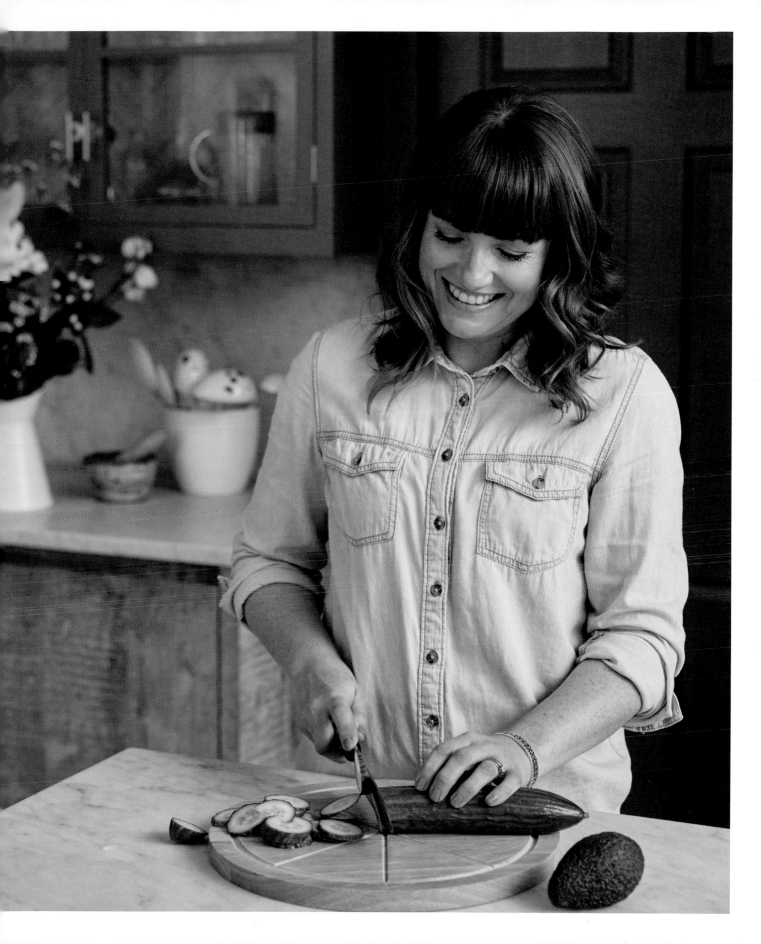

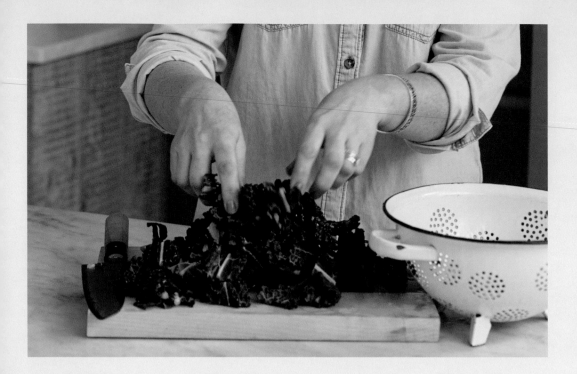

KEY NUTRIENTS FOR HEALTHY WEIGHT

B VITAMINS You need good levels of these vitamins to turn food into energy. A varied diet with a plentiful intake of vegetables, nuts and seeds, whole grains and some lean meat and fish should provide enough.

OMEGA 3 This is an "essential fat", so called because we can't manufacture it within the body and it is essential for pretty much every cell. High circulating blood sugar has been linked to low omega 3 fats because cells become resistant to insulin, a major factor in weight gain and type 2 diabetes. Omega 3 is found predominantly in oily fish (tinned is an excellent source and sometimes better than fresh), walnuts, chia seeds, hemp and flaxseed.

ZINC Important to control sugar cravings and general appetite control, this mineral plays an important role in the production of thyroid hormones. It is found in nuts and seeds, particularly pumpkin, and shellfish.

CHROMIUM Helps to balance blood sugar to prevent the highs and lows that can bring about food cravings and overeating of refined carbohydrates and sugar.

It's difficult to get enough of this mineral from diet alone because it's destroyed with cooking so a supplement of 200 mcg of chromium picolinate a day can be useful.

PROBIOTICS These are defined by the World Health Organization as "live microorganisms which when administered in adequate amounts, confer a health benefit on the host". Find them in yogurt and fermented foods such as miso and natto, kimchee, saukeraut and kefir.

VITAMIN D A staggering 50 percent of adults in the northern hemisphere are deficient in vitamin D, which we need for healthy bones. The body makes this vitamin when skin is exposed to sunlight (SPF has a blocking effect). We only get around 15 percent of vitamin D from our diet (egg yolks and oily fish), but it is important to test your levels before supplementing to get the dose right – because it is fat-soluble, vitamin D can store in the liver rather than being excreted. The optimal level in blood is 100–120nmol/l. It's best to take a liquid form.

STORE CUPBOARD ESSENTIALS

TINNED TOMATOES perfect as a base for spaghetti bolognaise, stews, curries and soups.

PULSES great source of vegetable protein, zinc, calcium and magnesium. Choose from chickpeas, lentils (Puy, red, green, beluga, brown, continental), butter beans, borlotti, cannellini, flageolet, kidney and black beans. Tins or pouches are easy to use.

BROWN RICE converts into sugar at a slower rate than white rice and is full of B vitamins and zinc, unlike its white counterpart.

NUTS AND SEEDS great source of protein, essential fats and zinc, and perfect for snacking.

WHOLEMEAL PASTA breaks down into sugar at a slower rate than regular pasta.

NATURAL YOGURT choose full-fat versions (Greek-style is only 8–10 percent fat) so you keep blood-sugar levels stable and feel fuller for longer. Avoid fruit yogurt; even small pots can contain up to 7 teaspoons of sugar.

HUMMUS select full-fat, which is full of protein, fibre and healthy monounsaturated fats.

OLIVES packed with healthy monounsaturated fats.

FISH fresh is usually best, but tinned is incredibly nutritious and cheap. Oily fish provides a good amount of protein and omega 3 fats, and tinned fish containing bones is an excellent source of calcium.

EGGS preferably organic or at least free range. Eggs are rich in vitamins A and D and a great source of protein. They do not increase cholesterol, so enjoy freely.

TOFU great vegetarian protein providing hormone-balancing phytoestrogens. Have fun with it.

QUINOA a pseudo-grain which is mainly protein and rich in B vitamins and zinc.

MEAT choose lean cuts, preferably organic or at least free range. Have a minimum two meat-free meals a week. Try adding Puy or green lentils to mince so it goes further and has more plant protein. Or throw red lentils into chicken curry, which do the same while naturally thickening the sauce

CHEESE eat a variety and avoid low-fat. Goat's cheese is more digestible.

COCONUT OIL gets a bad rep as a saturated fat, but its specific medium-chain fatty acids boost thermogenesis, heat production in the body that increases your metabolic rate. Studies show it has a positive effect on cholesterol. It also contains lauric acid and caprylic acid, which are naturally anti-microbial and anti-fungal.

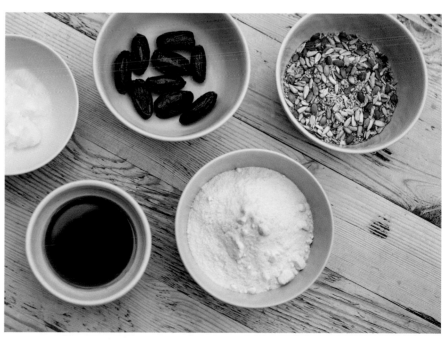

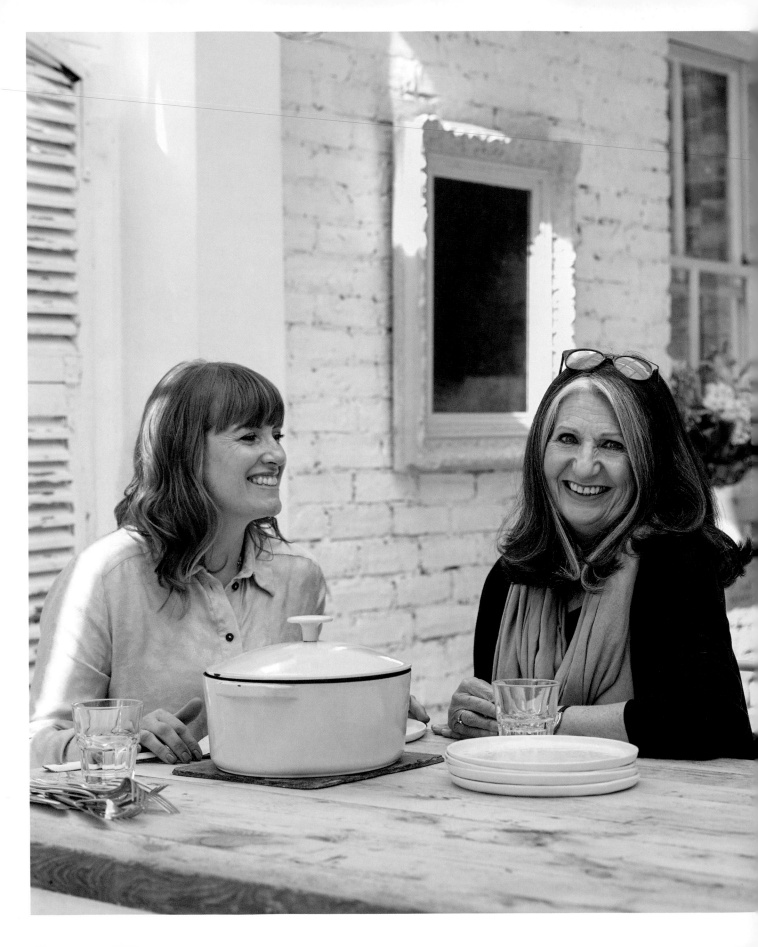

TOP FOOD TIPS

• If you are not doing 16/8 fasting, start the day with breakfast, preferably within an hour of waking to stop the spike in adrenaline and cortisol.

• Eat regular meals – every 3 hours – to keep blood sugar stable.

• Have protein with every meal and snack – add ground nuts or seeds to porridge, for example. This slows the conversion of carbohydrates into sugar to maintain energy levels and keep you fuller for longer.

• Keep wheat to a minimum – the way it is grown means it has high levels of gluten (protein) which can irritate the gut, and mineral-deficient soils can lead to a loss of nutrients. Clinical experience suggests many people without an intolerance or allergy feel better on a low-wheat diet.

• Do not count calories – it is not sustainable and not all calories are treated equally by the body.

• Throw away scales – they are soul-destroying, demotivating and create obsessive behaviour.

• Don't feel the need to cook complicated masterpieces – aim for good food from fresh ingredients.

• Menu plan – it really helps to know what you will be eating each week.

• Shop online to save on impulse buys and plan meals more efficiently.

• Eat more plant foods – build up from one meat-free meal a week.

• Avoid diet foods – there is always a catch, usually added sweeteners, and a list of ingredients your great-grandmother wouldn't recognize as food.

• Avoid fruit juice, or dilute it. When you eat a whole apple the sugars break down slowly because of the fibre; removing the skin and flesh leaves only fruit

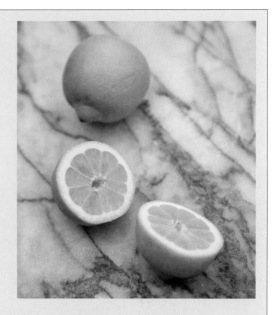

sugar in liquid form. This hits the bloodstream quickly, causing the release of insulin.

• Make your own flavoured water by freezing cubes of ginger, cucumber, lime and mint.

• Halve your current intake of alcohol. Avoiding it altogether may not be sustainable long term, but have at least three alcohol-free nights a week.

• Choose herbal teas and limit tea and coffee to one a day. They stress the adrenal glands and spike blood-sugar levels.

• Avoid artificial sweeteners – 100 times sweeter than sugar, they increase cravings and regular consumers have been shown to have larger waist circumferences. Research suggests they damage the gut microbiome (see page 28).

• Take your time. Plans that promise quick fixes and rapid weight loss can't be sustained and risk trapping you on a yo-yo dieting cycle.

• Don't be hard on yourself. It can take a good six months to work out what is right for you and change ingrained habits.

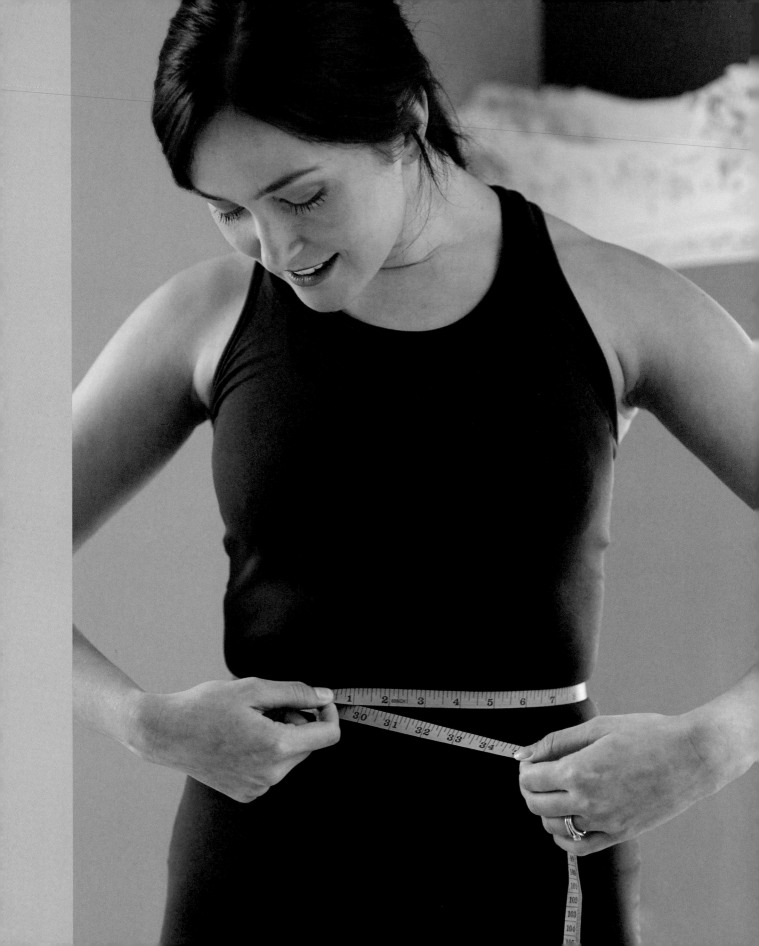

WEIGHT
Management

We've already discussed the importance of making the right lifestyle choices for our optimum health and wellbeing. Let's look now at weight again in more depth.

In spite of the rise of gym culture, the drive toward clean eating and an endless stream of health articles, wellness blogs and government-driven media campaigns, the problem of obesity is increasing around the world.

In February 2018, the World Health Organization (WHO) stated that worldwide obesity had nearly tripled since 1975, with 39 percent of adults overweight in 2016 and 13 percent obese. Most of the world's population now live in countries where being overweight and obese kills more people than being underweight. Being obese can increase your risk of developing many potentially serious health conditions, from type 2 diabetes, high blood pressure, asthma and osteoarthritis to reduced fertility and pregnancy complications. Obesity reduces life expectancy by an average of 3–10 years. And yet it is preventable.

According to WHO, the fundamental cause of obesity and being overweight is the energy imbalance between calories consumed and calories expended. We believe this is part of the equation but not the full picture. Worldwide, in recent years we have seen an increased intake of energy-dense foods that are high in fat, with a rise also in physical inactivity due to the increasingly sedentary nature of many forms of work, changing modes of transport and growing urbanization. Obesity is about much more than the rise in portion size and the wrong type of food on our plates.

ADDITIONAL HEALTH PROBLEMS ASSOCIATED WITH OBESITY

- Breathlessness.
- Increased sweating.
- Snoring.
- Difficulty doing physical activity.
- Joint and back pain.
- Low confidence and self-esteem.
- Feeling isolated.

Do genes play a role? According to Giles Yeo, Principal Research Associate at the University of Cambridge Neuroscience Community in the UK, there is a close link between our genes and our weight. Yeo writes, in his book *Gene Eating*, that certain peoples, for example the Pima peoples in Arizona and Pacific Islanders, are among the heaviest in the world. Their obesity, he explains, is linked to the evolution of genes that helped them survive harsh conditions and times of famine. The problem is that their bodies have not adjusted when food is plentiful. Obese people, he argues, are "fighting their biology". We cannot control our genes, but thankfully there are aspects of life we can control, from sleep to stress management, that can help us become healthier and fitter.

Achieving your optimum weight
– how to get started

Before we begin, you first need to work out if you need to lose weight and if so, how much. You may just simply want to tone up. And what actually is a successful weight-loss programme?

Scales are useful but can be deceptive. How your clothes fit is a better guide to where you put on weight – is your waistband tight, do jeans slide easily over your hips, do jumpers feel tight around your arms and shoulders?

Then stand in front of a mirror holding a small mirror. Look at yourself from 360 degrees. Are there areas that need a little help? Be honest, but not harsh or judgemental. Your body works very hard for you and deserves respect.

Now, if it's helpful, work out and record your Body Mass Index (BMI) and hip-to-waist ratio (see opposite and page 38). This can help to motivate you, especially if you find yourself plateauing (a common experience) as the weeks pass, by reminding you of what you have already achieved.

According to 2005 research in *The American Journal of Clinical Nutrition*, a successful weight-loss programme is one where at least 10 percent of weight is intentionally lost and the new weight maintained for at least a year.

BODY COMPOSITION

There are several methods to measure total body fat. The most accurate is a bioelectrical impedance scale, a device using electrical currents to determine fat levels. But the most common method used globally by doctors and fitness professionals to assess if weight is putting health at risk is the Body Mass Index (BMI). BMI doesn't give information about body fat, so for a better idea of

"It won't be the easiest of journeys …
but then the ones worth making
never are." ANON

how much weight you need to lose it's best combined with your waist-to-hip circumference ratio (see page 38).

Our bodies are made up of two components: lean body mass (LBM) and fat. Lean body mass consists of organs such as the heart, liver, pancreas, bones, skin and, of course, muscle tissue. All need oxygen and nutrients from food in order to grow and for repair. Muscle, in particular, has a high metabolic rate and burns calories quickly. Fat does not need oxygen, does not repair itself and has a low metabolic rate, so doesn't burn calories.

We all need some body fat for warmth, insulation and normal organic functions. Having too little body fat carries its own health risks – the decreased fertility associated with amenorrhea (when menstruation ceases), which may also affect the long-term health of bones. There is a lot of pressure on all of us, but young girls in particular, to stay slim. Sadly, this can contribute to eating disorders such as anorexia nervosa and bulimia. If you think you may have an eating disorder or feel afraid to put on weight, please consult your medical practitioner.

The ratio of lean body mass to fat is important. Your lean body mass is constantly altering because of changes in your muscles. People with a low lean body mass often lack energy and risk muscle degeneration and premature ageing. This is a very good reason for avoiding slimming diets. On faddish diets with no

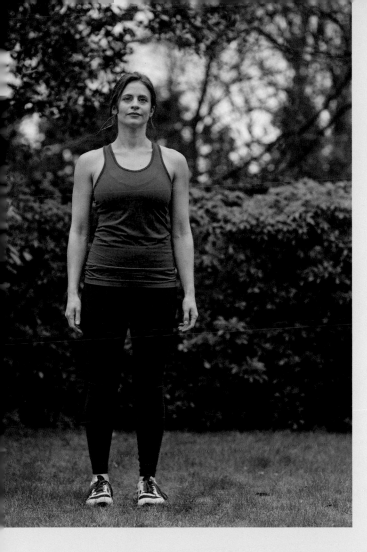

exercise you will shed lean muscle tissue, which causes your body to lose muscle tone and your energy levels to drop.

A BMI may give a "false" reading for athletes with lots of muscle. A pound of muscle tissue weighs the same as a pound of fat, but muscle tissue takes up less space, which is why the guy with the six-pack might weigh the same as the guy with the beer belly – but the six-pack guy's jeans fit better! BMI is also not accurate during pregnancy or if you are breastfeeding or if you are very frail.

The way to streamline your body, improve your energy levels, boost your immune system and achieve optimum health lies in increasing your lean body mass with exercise and a healthy balanced diet.

HOW TO CALCULATE YOUR BODY MASS INDEX (BMI)

BMI = your weight (in kilograms) / your height (in metres) squared
Example: 60kg/ (1.65m x 1.65m) = 22
1kg = 2.2lb 1m = 39.37in

MY BMI
Date

READING THE SCORES

BMI BELOW 18.5 – CONSIDERED UNDERWEIGHT
You may need to gain weight for health reasons. Consult your doctor if you have concerns or feel afraid to put on weight.

BMI OF 18.5–25 – NORMAL
For health reasons you need to stay in this range. You may lose some weight for appearance, and you may need to tone up.

BMI OF 25–30 – OVERWEIGHT
You should lose some weight for health reasons.

BMI OF 30–40 – OBESE
Your health is at risk, and losing weight will improve your health.

BMI OF OVER 40 – MORBIDLY OBESE
Your health is seriously at risk, and you should visit your doctor.

Waist-to-hip ratio – apple or pear?

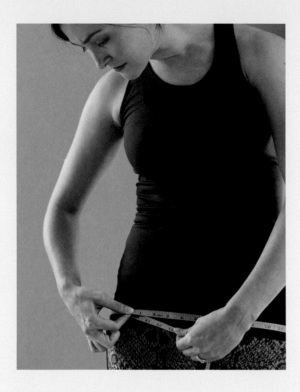

Storing fat may have been a lifesaver for our ancestors. When food was scarce, we stored body fat to boost the immune system and prevent infection. However, for most of us, food is now readily available and this process of storing fat has serious health implications.

Fat stored around the waist has been linked with health problems, particularly an increased risk of type 2 diabetes, heart disease, high blood pressure and abnormal blood-fat levels. In women, this "central" obesity, which creates a typically apple-shaped figure, is also associated with a higher risk of pre-menopausal breast cancer. Fat stored around the hips, creating a typical pear shape, seems less problematic.

So while the waist-to-hip ratio does not give the full picture, it does indicate whether we have an increased health risk. And in the meantime, we can take action by increasing physical activity and eating healthily.

HOW TO MEASURE YOUR WAIST-TO-HIP RATIO

Use a standard tape measure.

1 WAIST
Stand tall, but relax your waist (do not cheat by pulling your tummy in). Locate the narrowest point of your waist (normally around the navel) and measure around.

MY WAIST MEASUREMENT
Date

2 HIP
Still standing tall, find the widest point of your hips and buttocks and measure around.

MY HIP MEASUREMENT
Date

3 WAIST-TO-HIP RATIO.
Divide the results from 1 (waist) by the results from 2 (hip). This gives your waist-to-hip ratio.

MY WAIST-TO-HIP RATIO
Date

EXAMPLE
Waist measurement: 75cm (30in)
Hip measurement: 92.5cm (37in)
Waist-to-hip ratio: 75 / 92.5 = 0.80

READING THE SCORES
WOMEN aim for a waist-to-hip ratio of less than 0.80.
MEN aim for a waist-to-hip ratio of less than 0.90.

So you need to lose weight?

If your BMI and waist-to-hip ratio suggest you are overweight, record the results, along with your weight and height in a notebook or on your phone, computer or fitness tracker.

Health professionals encourage us to aim for 5–10 percent weight loss over 3–6 months. How does this translate? If you weigh 80kg (176lb), a healthy weight loss over six months would be around 8kg (17.5lb). Your goal weight would be 72kg (158lb).

The ideal rate of weight loss you should aim for to remain healthy is around 0.5–1kg (1–2lb) per week. If this sounds very slow, bear three things in mind:

1   This is about healthy weight loss and optimum health. Be wary of weight-loss plans that promise dramatic results in a few weeks.
2   As muscle tissue replaces fat, but weighs more, scales are not the best judge of progress.
3   Your body shape will change noticeably. You will lose inches and look more toned and streamlined.

If your BMI score classifies you as overweight, your goal is to bring your score into the "normal" category (see page 37). Similarly, if your waist-to-hip ratio was over the norm (see opposite), aim to bring it within recommended guidelines.

Once you have achieved this, you may continue to improve your fitness and sculpt your body, but please do not allow your BMI or body-fat measurement (if you have this tested) to drop below what is considered normal. Retest and record your scores regularly, say every two weeks, while following this programme.

Keep a record of your progress and take note if you think of ways to achieve your goals. Writing everything down helps clarify things and highlights weaknesses

and strengths. Revisit your personal record every fortnight to see how your weight, waist-to-hip ratio and BMI are changing. But please bear in mind that none gives the full picture of achievements. Your jeans may tell you more!

Take things slowly if you are out of condition. Remember, you do not have to complete the Shape Up programme within 12 weeks.

SETTING REALISTIC GOALS

Planning in advance is essential to success with Pilates, cardio activities, weight loss and changes to your diet.

- Note in your diary when you will train and stick to it.
- If commitments prevent you from doing the full 150 minutes of Pilates one week, work out how much time you can spare. Any more is a bonus.
- Do not give up if you fail to meet goals. Even small progress is progress.
- Give yourself a target, such as a holiday, wedding or school reunion.
- When you reach the target, take stock and plan for another event.

The Shape Up programme – how it works

To achieve the goal of a new body in three months, we would like you – ideally – to do approximately 150 minutes (2½ hours) of Pilates a week. You don't need a stop watch, it doesn't have to be that precise.

You choose how often and how long to work out each week. You can vary the length of workouts to, say, 7 x 20 minutes one week and 3 x 45 minutes the next – you just need to keep track of timings.

All the workouts are perfectly balanced except the 10-minute workouts (which are as balanced as they can be). If you do both 10-minute mini workouts in a day, you'll have a balanced workout too.

If you miss your 150-minute weekly goal, don't panic. This isn't an exact equation, so just do a little extra the following week. If 150 minutes isn't doable, do as much as you can, bearing in mind that it may take a little longer to get results.

As you get further into the programme, feel free to mix and match the workouts. For example, you could add a 30-minute workout to a 10-minute one, or add two 30-minute workouts together. Just leave out any duplicate exercises.

If you are concerned with one area of your body – perhaps your upper arms, tummy, thighs or bottom – turn to the relevant Shape Up Even More pages (see pages 114–185) for specific exercises targeting those areas. To be honest, this goes against our Pilates' philosophy because your whole body is involved in every Pilates exercise. But it's fair to say that each Shape Up Even More exercise targets one part of the body a little more than the rest.

ADDING IT UP

To reach the goal of roughly 150 minutes of Pilates a week you can opt for:

- 14 x 10 minutes (daily mini-workouts, am and pm)
- 5 x 30 minutes
- 3 x 45–50 minutes

BEFORE YOU BEGIN

Please check with your doctor that it is safe for you to exercise before starting a new programme, especially if you have a health condition. Only your doctor knows your full medical history – for example, if hypothyroidism is causing weight gain, no amount of exercise or dieting will help until it is under control. Our books *The Pilates Bible* and *Pilates for Life* give specific guidance on exercising for the heart, bone health and other common conditions.

Everything you need to know for good Pilates practice is contained within this book.

Here we will share with you some exercise tips we've learnt from years of teaching experience. When you've digested this section, start with the New Fundamentals chapter even if you have done Pilates before. Even the most experienced Pilates teacher revisits them regularly, and we constantly update our teaching. We have built exercise combinations and sequences from these Fundamentals, so you need to know them. We know you want a new body in three months, but getting the Fundamental exercises right guarantees that you get

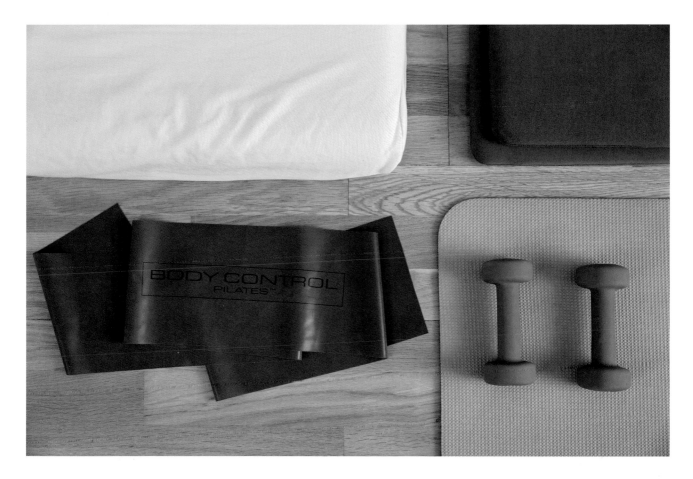

the most from your workouts. It's like reading a recipe before starting to cook.

Alongside the New Fundamentals are Shape Up More exercises showing ways to increase the toning power. Each exercise also has a level of difficulty from 1–6, with 1 being the easiest and 6 the most challenging.

SHAPE UP MORE

It's very important not to try the Shape Up More exercises until you are familiar with the basic versions and strong and flexible enough to do them well. To help, we've provided workouts solely made up of Fundamental exercises (see pages 197–199). When you've mastered these, try the workouts mixing exercises from levels 1–2, 2–3 and so on, gradually building your movement skills, strength and flexibility.

EQUIPMENT

- Padded non-slip mat.
- Folded towel or small flat pillow.
- Firm bed pillow.
- Medium-strength, long stretch band, or a long, stretchy scarf.
- Sturdy chair.
- Always practise without weights first. Then choose light weights (under 0.5kg/1.1lb each weight). Only increase the weight if good technique is guaranteed.

TIPS FOR GOOD PRACTICE

- Prepare your exercise space by making it warm, comfortable and free from distraction.

- Make sure you have enough room to move your arms and legs freely.

- If you use music, try to play it quietly so that it is not distracting.

- Wear clothing that allows for freedom of movement but also lets you see your alignment.

- Barefoot is best, but you can wear non-slip socks. If exercising outdoors, try to wear flexible, thin-soled shoes.

- Remember the ABCs of Alignment, Breathing and Centring (see page 46) at all times.

- Check the level of difficulty of an exercise before practising: 1 is for beginners, 6 advanced.

- Work at your own pace and move on to more challenging versions of exercises only when you are ready (remember that some Starting Positions up the level of difficulty).

- Read each exercise carefully and note its main focus, perhaps the area of the body targeted or a movement skill.

- Take time to find the correct Starting Alignment (see pages 48–61) to enhance the precision of your movements. If your Starting Position isn't right, your movements won't be right.

- Before trying a Shape Up More version of a Fundamental exercise, make sure you can do the simpler version well and check the level of difficulty.

- Make sure you understand all the movements described in the Action Points, checking against the photographs.

- Use the Watchpoints for tips on honing your technique and avoiding common pitfalls. You might find it helpful to check your alignment initially in a mirror.

- Value quality over number of repetitions. We give the ideal number or reps for muscle-building results. But if your technique is suffering because your muscles are fatiguing, stop and rest.

- Start with a different leg, arm or side each time you practise. We all favour one side, so balance this out.

- Start and end one-legged or one-armed exercises with a repetition on two limbs, for balance.

- Return to the Starting Position with control after each repetition and at the end of the sequence – this is as important as the exercise itself.

- Do some Deep Abdominal Breathing (page 62) before and after your session.

- When practising exercises or sequences combining two movements, practise the movements separately for a few repetitions, to maintain quality.

- Do not be tempted to speed up the exercises. This may increase the aerobic quality of the exercises but does not affect the toning power.

- Slow exercises down to challenge yourself. With Pilates it's important to sweat the small stuff.

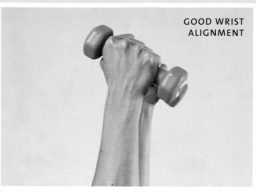

GOOD WRIST
ALIGNMENT

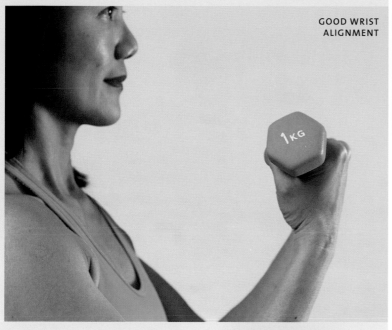

GOOD WRIST
ALIGNMENT

USING WEIGHTS SAFELY

- Maintain good wrist alignment (see the photographs above and left).

- Practise first without weights, then gradually increase the weight over time.

- Do not increase the weight at the expense of good technique. For some exercises, we suggest using the lightest weights.

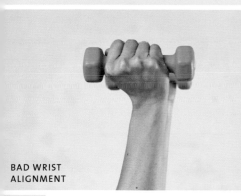

BAD WRIST
ALIGNMENT

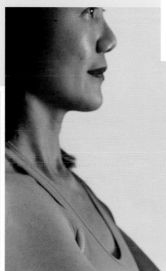

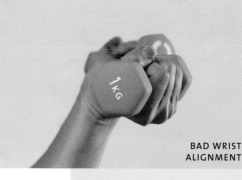

BAD WRIST
ALIGNMENT

WHEN NOT TO EXERCISE

- If you feel unwell.

- After a heavy meal or drinking alcohol.

- If you are in pain from injury (consult a healthcare practitioner, who may advise rest).

- If taking strong painkillers (which can mask warning signs).

- When undergoing medical treatment or taking medication (consult your medical practitioner before starting a programme).

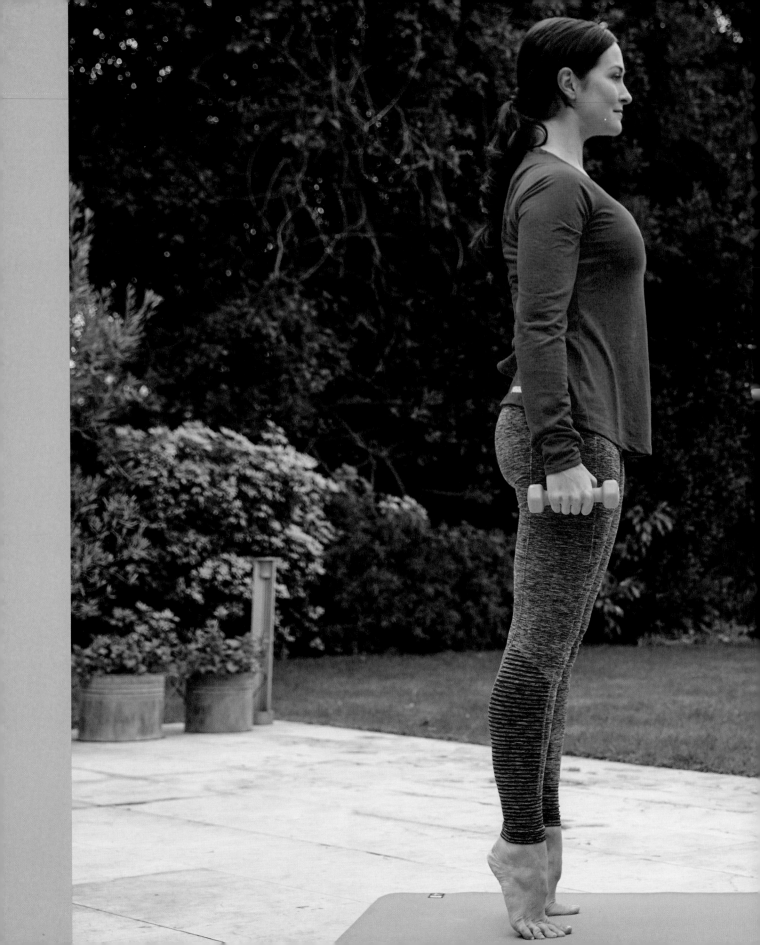

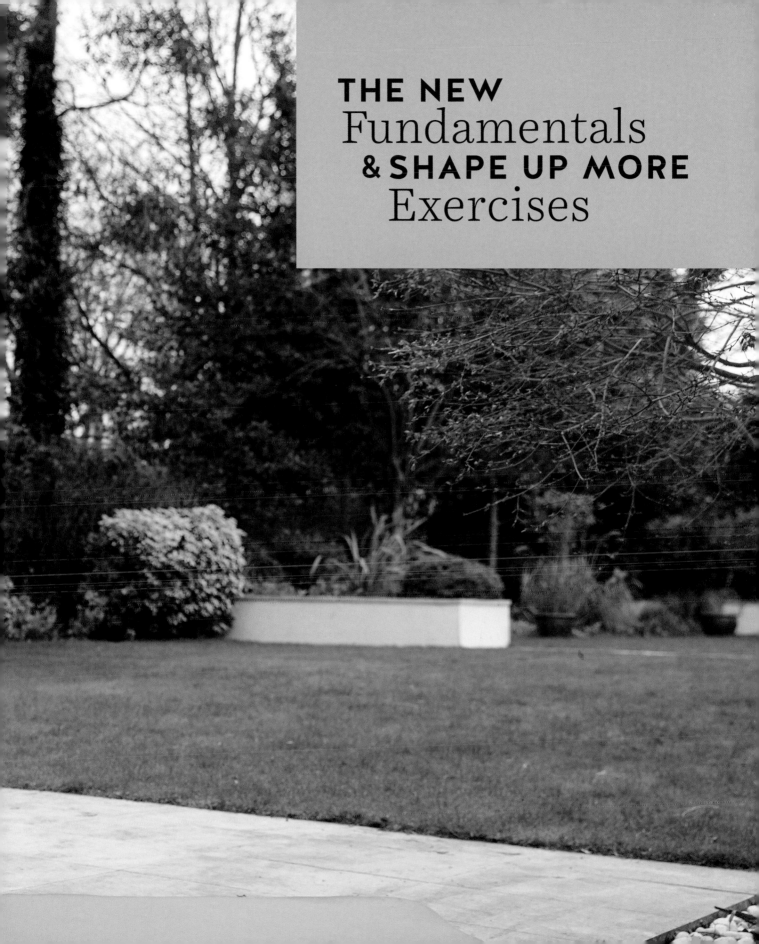

THE NEW
Fundamentals
& SHAPE UP MORE
Exercises

Alignment

"Controlology [Pilates] ... is designed to give you suppleness, natural grace and skill that will be unmistakeably reflected in the way you walk, in the way you play, and in the way you work."

JOSEPH PILATES

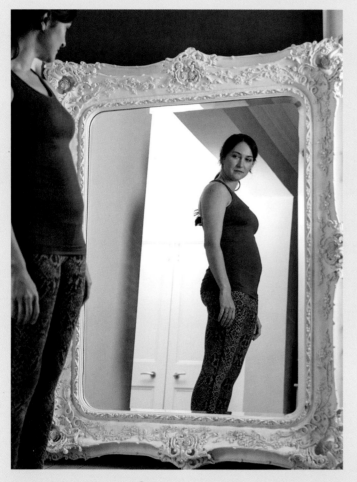

Poor posture is very unflattering.

This is, without question, the most important section of the book – skip it at your peril! These New Fundamentals will ensure not only that you are working correctly, but that you get the maximum benefit from the exercises. Try not to think of the ABCs of Alignment, Breathing and Centring as being just for beginners. They have to be incorporated into every move you make.

But first let's put them in context. The ABCs are taken from Body Control Pilates' Eight Principles. These underpin our whole approach.

1 Concentration
2 Relaxation
3 Alignment
4 Breathing
5 Centring
6 Co-ordination
7 Flowing Movements
8 Stamina

The areas that we will be focusing on in this chapter are how to find good postural Alignment in a variety of positions, how to Breathe efficiently during the exercises and how to stay Centred while you move.

Good alignment is fundamental to good practice. How you start and finish exercises and your control of alignment while performing them, will make a big difference to how effective they are.

Good postural alignment can also make a difference to how you look and gives you what Joseph Pilates called "graceful carriage".

Try this experiment. Stand in front of a mirror and slouch (as in the photo on the page opposite). What do you see?

· Your stomach sticks out
· Your waist disappears as your ribs sink toward your hips
· You appear shorter

Try the same experiment but standing tall. Elongate your spine by lengthening through the crown of your head. Open your shoulders, allowing your arms to relax down by your sides. For a moment, gently draw your lower abdominals back toward your spine. Breathe. Observe the changes:

· You look instantly taller
· You have given your breasts a lift
· Your waist has reappeared
· Your stomach looks flatter
· Notice too how you feel better in yourself

The problem is that for most of us standing tall is very tiring, requiring enormous inner strength from your deep postural muscles. The deep "core" muscles are anti-gravity muscles. When they are weak it is very difficult to maintain good posture all day.

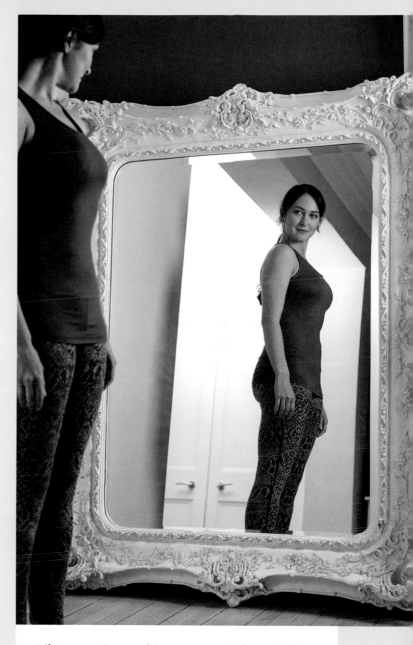

Pilates can give you this core strength from within, and the ability to stand tall without effort day in, day out. This natural grace and elegance has drawn stage performers and dancers to Pilates for decades. But there is more to good posture than alignment of the bones and strong core muscles. You have to feel good posture, understand it and experience it. This section will help you do that not just during the exercises, but for life.

STARTING POSITIONS

These are the Starting and Finishing Positions for the exercises in the book. If they aren't right, then you will not be moving correctly. There are seated, kneeling, prone, side-lying and standing positions, and you will find different head, arm and leg positions used throughout the book, which can change the level of difficulty. The easiest position to learn good alignment is Relaxation Position because the ground gives feedback, helping you feel what is correct.

RELAXATION POSITION LEVEL 1

This is an exercise in itself as well as the start and finish position for many lying exercises. As an exercise, use Relaxation Position to release unwanted tension and improve body awareness for good postural alignment, breathing and stability. As a Starting Position, use it to check your ABCs before moving. If resting in this position, use additional props for comfort (remove before starting an exercise).

STARTING POSITION

Lie on your back on the mat with knees bent, feet hip-width apart and in parallel. Aim your heels toward the centre of each buttock to find hip-width apart.

If required, place a small folded towel or firm flat pillow beneath your head. The neck should be lengthened but maintain its natural "cervical" curve and neither tip forward nor back. Some people don't need a pillow, others may need two.

STARTING POSITION

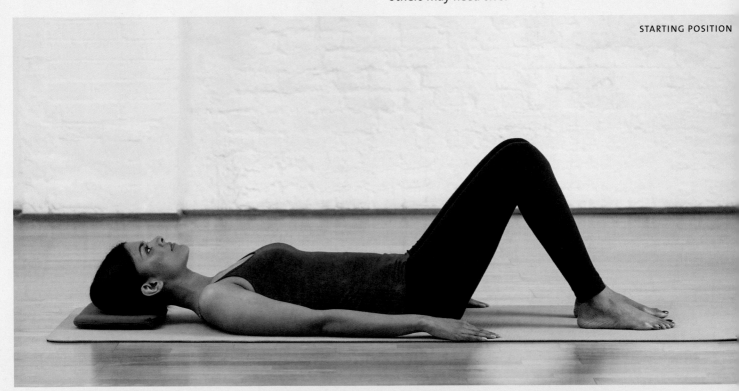

ACTION

If remaining in Relaxation Position, place your hands on your lower abdomen to allow your shoulders to widen and open.

If using Relaxation Position as a Starting Position for another exercise, relax your arms by your sides, palms facing the floor.

To come out, roll onto your side and rest for a moment before sitting up.

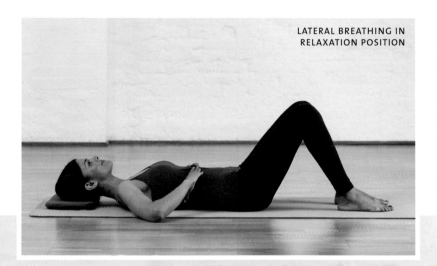

LATERAL BREATHING IN
RELAXATION POSITION

WATCHPOINTS

➜ Allow your entire spine to widen and lengthen, feel supported by the mat.

➜ Focus on three areas of body weight: your ribcage, pelvis and head.

➜ Allow your thighs to sink toward your hips and your lower legs toward your ankles; let your feet be grounded.

➜ Focus on width across your chest, release in the breastbone.

➜ Allow your neck to feel lengthened, your jaw released.

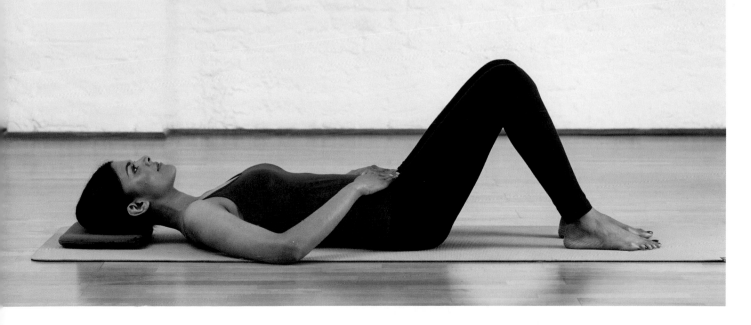

CHECKING NEUTRAL
AND CONNECTING
TO YOUR CORE

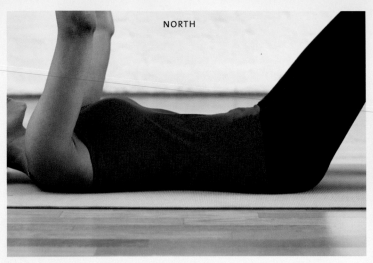

NORTH

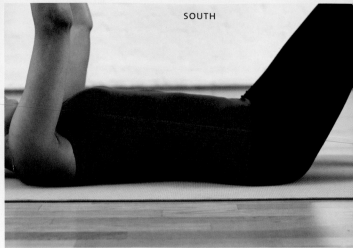

SOUTH

THE COMPASS LEVEL 1

Designed to help you develop an awareness of neutral alignment around the pelvis and lower spine, this exercise is also a great way to mobilize and release the lower back.

STARTING POSITION

Relaxation Position (see page 48), lengthening your arms by your sides. Imagine a compass on your lower abdomen; your navel is north, your pubic bone south and the prominent bones of your pelvis on either side west and east.

ACTION

1 Breathe in to prepare.
2 Breathe out as you gently tilt your pelvis north (the pubic bone moves forward and up). Feel your lower spine release into the mat as your pelvis tilts backward.
3 Breathe in as you tilt your pelvis back through the mid-position without stopping until the pelvis tilts gently forward to the south (the pubic bone moves backward and down). Your lower back will arch slightly.

Repeat this north/south tilt 5 times.

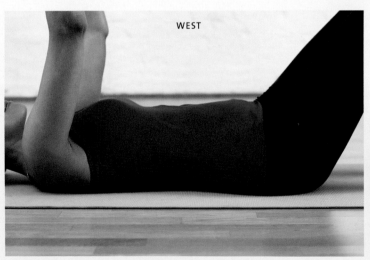

WEST

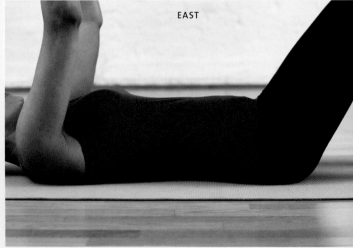

EAST

WATCHPOINTS

➜ Use appropriate core connection to control your alignment and movements (see pages 64–65).

➜ The tilting and final neutral position should feel comfortable.

➜ In neutral, feel the back of your pelvis (sacrum) heavy and grounded into the mat.

➜ Check that your waist is equally lengthened on both sides.

➜ Ensure there is equal weight on both sides of the pelvis.

➜ Allow your hip joints to be free.

➜ Once you have found your neutral pelvis, remember the rest of the body. Run through all the Watchpoints for Relaxation Position (page 49).

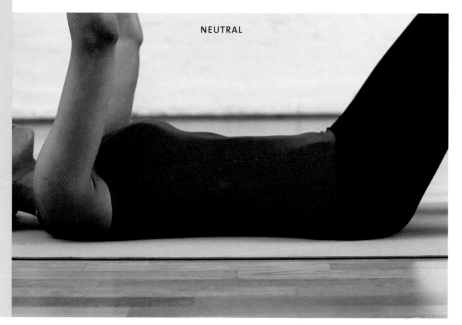

NEUTRAL

4 Now return to the Starting Position and find your neutral position, the mid-position neither north nor south but in between.

5 Breathe out as you roll your pelvis to one side – west. Feel the opposite side of the pelvis lift slightly as the pelvis rotates. Try to roll directly to the side without shortening one side of your waist (hip-hiking).

6 Breathe in as you roll your pelvis through the mid-position, without stopping, to the other side – east. Feel the opposite side of your pelvis lift slightly as your pelvis rotates.

7 Return to the mid-position (neither east, west, north nor south but in between). Your pelvis is level. This is your neutral position.

8 To come out, roll onto your side and rest for a moment before sitting up.

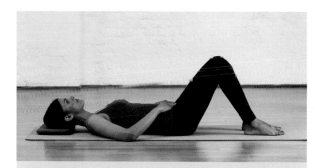

QUICK NEUTRAL CHECK

Place your hands on your lower abdomen, making a triangular shape. Your fingers touch your pubic bone and the base of your thumbs rest on your prominent pelvic bones. When you are in neutral, your hands are parallel to the floor (tummy permitting) and both sides of your waist are equal in length.

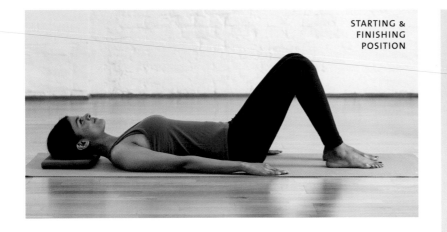

STARTING & FINISHING POSITION

WATCHPOINTS

➜ The movements should feel natural and comfortable.

➜ Keep your neck long throughout.

➜ As you draw your chin down, in the tuck action, the back of your head slides up the mat (don't press the back of your neck into the mat).

➜ Try not to disturb the natural neutral curves of your upper and lower back.

CHIN TUCKS AND NECK ROLLS LEVEL 1

Like the Compass, this exercise will help your awareness of neutral alignment around your head and neck. You roll the head through different positions, coming to rest in a neutral mid-position. It's also a really effective way to release tension in the neck and is perfect for any warm-up phase of a workout. The Chin Tuck action is used a lot when doing abdominal exercises like Curl Ups (page 92).

STARTING POSITION

Relaxation Position (page 48), lengthening your arms by your sides on the mat.

ACTION: CHIN TUCK

1 Breathe in to prepare.

2 Breathe out as you lengthen the back of your neck, nodding your head forward, drawing the chin down. Keep your head in contact with the mat.

3 Breathe in as you tip your head back gently, passing through the mid-position without stopping, to slightly extend your neck. Once again keep the back of the head in contact with the mat as the chin glides upward; this is a small movement.

4 Repeat 5 times, then find the mid-position where your head is neither tipped back or forward. Your neck should now be in neutral, with your face and focus directed toward the ceiling.

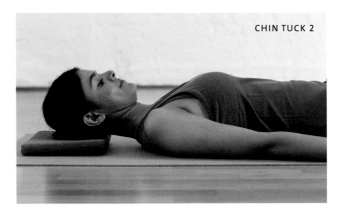

CHIN TUCK 2

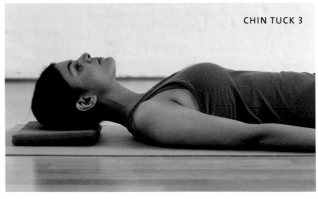

CHIN TUCK 3

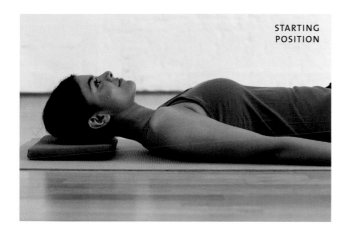

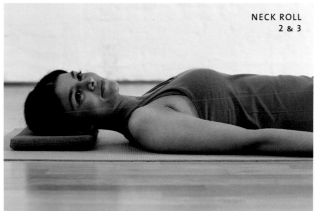

ACTION: NECK ROLLS

1 Breathe out as you roll your head to one side.
Again, keep your head in contact with the mat.
2 Breathe in as you roll your head back to centre.
3 Repeat to the other side, then repeat the Neck Roll up
to 5 times before returning your head back to centre
with even length on both sides of your neck.

SEATED ON A MAT (LONG FROG) LEVEL 1

Sit upright on the mat. You may feel more comfortable
sitting on a rolled-up towel or cushion to help the spine
into a neutral position. Bend your knees, turn your legs
out from the hips and connect the soles of your feet.
Have your feet a distance from the body to give a feeling
of space in the hip joints. Place your hands on your
shins, lengthening your arms, with elbows slightly bent.

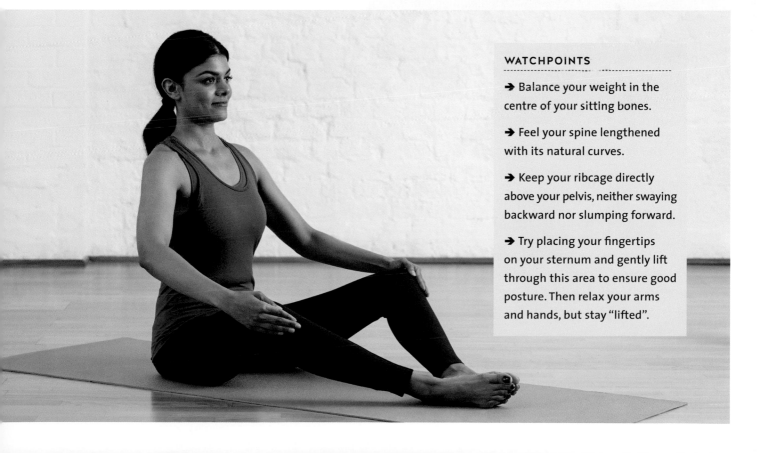

WATCHPOINTS

➜ Balance your weight in the
centre of your sitting bones.

➜ Feel your spine lengthened
with its natural curves.

➜ Keep your ribcage directly
above your pelvis, neither swaying
backward nor slumping forward.

➜ Try placing your fingertips
on your sternum and gently lift
through this area to ensure good
posture. Then relax your arms
and hands, but stay "lifted".

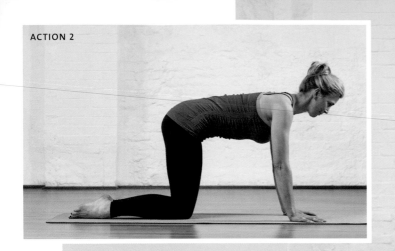

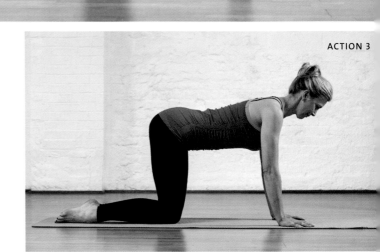

WATCHPOINTS

→ Use appropriate core connection to control your alignment and movements (see pages 64–65).

→ As with the Compass (page 50), the movements are subtle.

→ Fully lengthen your arms but do not lock your elbows.

→ Keep your chest and the front of your shoulders open and release any tension in your neck.

ACTION 3

FOUR-POINT KNEELING LEVEL 1

You cannot just rest in this position, you need to be active.

STARTING POSITION
Kneel on all fours on the mat. Position your hands directly beneath your shoulders and your knees directly beneath your hips.

ACTION: FINDING NEUTRAL PELVIS AND SPINE
1 Breathe in to prepare.
2 Breathe out as you tilt your pelvis backward (north, the pubic bone moves forward), allowing your lower back to slightly round (flex).

3 Breathe in and tilt your pelvis forward (south, your pubic bone moves backward), allowing your lower back to slightly arch (extend).
4 Repeat 3 times, then find the mid-position between these two extremes, where your pelvis is neutral. This position is lengthened and level, neither tucked nor arched and allows for the natural curvature of the lumbar spine.

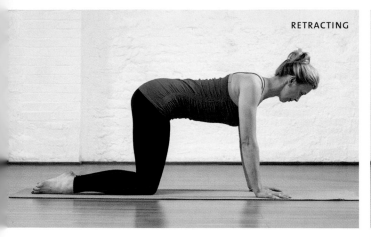
RETRACTING

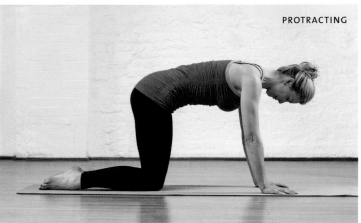
PROTRACTING

ACTION: FINDING GOOD SHOULDER ALIGNMENT

1 Breathe in and, keeping your elbows straight, gently draw your shoulder blades together (retracting them). Your upper spine will lower slightly toward the mat.

2 Breathe out as you allow your shoulder blades to glide wider on your ribcage (protracting them). Your upper spine will slightly round.

3 Repeat 3 times, then find the mid-position of the shoulder blades between these two extremes. Allow for the natural curvature of your upper spine and neck. Lengthen your whole spine from the crown of your head to your tailbone.

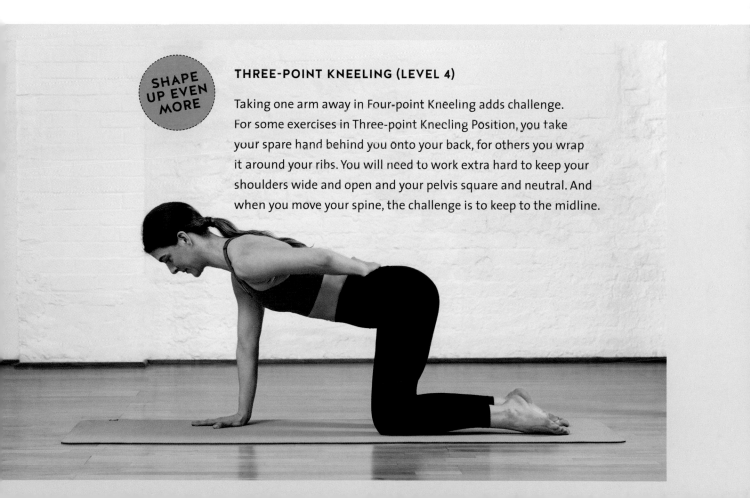

SHAPE UP EVEN MORE

THREE-POINT KNEELING (LEVEL 4)

Taking one arm away in Four-point Kneeling adds challenge. For some exercises in Three-point Kneeling Position, you take your spare hand behind you onto your back, for others you wrap it around your ribs. You will need to work extra hard to keep your shoulders wide and open and your pelvis square and neutral. And when you move your spine, the challenge is to keep to the midline.

➜ Use appropriate core connection to control your alignment and movements (see pages 64–65).

➜ Lengthen through your spine.

➜ Your ribcage is directly above your pelvis.

➜ Feel wide across your upper back and allow your collarbones to open.

➜ As before (page 53), try placing your fingertips on your sternum and gently lift through this area. Relax your hands, but stay lifted.

➜ Focus your gaze directly in front of you.

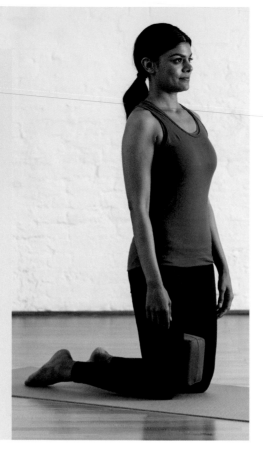

HIGH KNEELING (LEVEL 1)

You might prefer to practise on a padded mat to protect your knees, but not too padded or you will feel unstable. You can, if you wish, use a small cushion, about hip-width in thickness.

High kneel on your mat with knees hip-width apart. Place the cushion between your thighs (optional).

Check that your lower legs are parallel and hip-width apart, and that your weight drops not only through your knees, but evenly through the length of both shin bones.

HIGH KNEELING LUNGE POSITION (LEVEL 4)

Start by following the directions for High Kneeling (without the cushion), then bring one leg in front of you, in line with your hip. Make sure your bent knee is directly over your ankle so your knee is at a 90-degree angle. If you find this position uncomfortable, substitute High Kneeling instead.

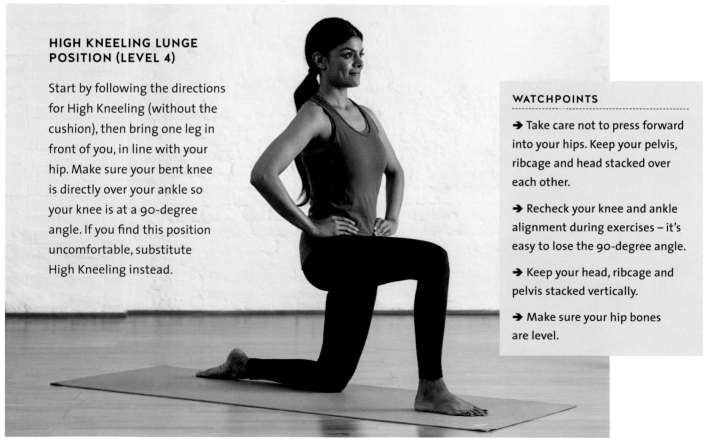

WATCHPOINTS

➜ Take care not to press forward into your hips. Keep your pelvis, ribcage and head stacked over each other.

➜ Recheck your knee and ankle alignment during exercises – it's easy to lose the 90-degree angle.

➜ Keep your head, ribcage and pelvis stacked vertically.

➜ Make sure your hip bones are level.

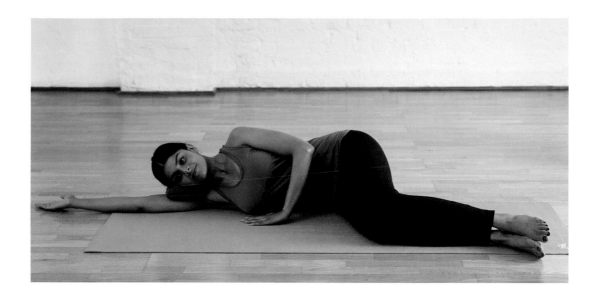

SIDE-LYING CHAIR POSITION (LEVEL 1)

There are different Side-lying Starting positions in the programme of varying levels of difficulty. This is the easiest. The harder positions reduce your base of support by, for example, having the legs straight in line with your body.

Lie on your side. Bend both knees in front of you so your hips and knees are bent at a right angle. Stack hip over hip, knee over knee, shoulder over shoulder. To check

you are straight, line up your torso with the back edge of your mat.

Stretch your underneath arm in line with your spine. Use a flat cushion or folded towel between your head and arm to keep your head aligned.

Bend your top arm, gently resting your hand in front of your torso for light support.

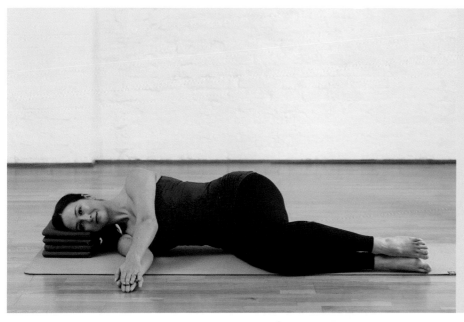

WATCHPOINTS

➜ Try to maintain the natural curves of the spine.

➜ Lengthen both sides of your waist equally; this is essential in side-lying as it is very easy for the lower side of your spine to dip toward the mat.

➜ In a side-lying exercise, such as Arm Openings (page 100), when your arms are in front of you, use enough head cushions to keep the head and neck aligned with the spine.

WATCHPOINTS

→ Use appropriate core connection to control your alignment and movements (see pages 64–65).

→ Your lower spine should feel lengthened. If there is any discomfort, place a flat folded towel beneath your abdomen to help support your spine.

→ Think of connecting the front of your lower ribcage and the top of your pelvis.

→ Allow your chest to open and your collarbones widen.

→ Keep your neck long; don't tuck in or lift your chin.

→ If you feel your legs might cramp, place a pillow under your shins.

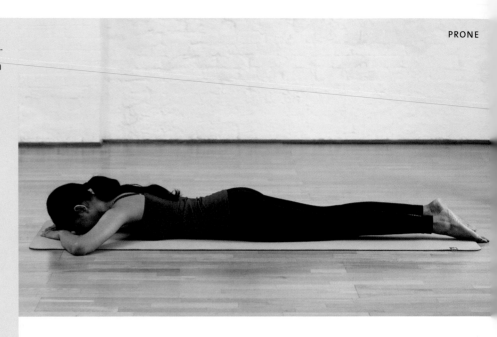

PRONE STARTING POSITION (LEVEL 1)

Here we have described one of the Prone Starting Positions. There are lots of variations.

Lie on your front and create a diamond shape with your arms.

Place your fingertips together, palms on the mat, and open your elbows. Rest your forehead on the backs of your hands. If it's more comfortable, widen your hands to allow your shoulders to broaden and relax (you may place a folded towel under your forehead). Place your legs hip-width apart and parallel.

STANDING IN PARALLEL (LEVEL 1)

Standing tall 24/7 means recruiting many of the body's deep postural muscles, the ones holding you up against gravity. Practice builds endurance – standing tall is a dynamic exercise rather than a "position" and requires you to be active, with 80 percent of your body weight balanced over the arches of your feet. We offer 18 Action Points to help you achieve this.

STARTING POSITION
Stand tall on the floor (not a mat) with feet hip-width apart in a natural stance, neither turned out nor in a rigid parallel position. Lengthen your arms by the sides of your body.

ACTION
1 Lean forward slightly from your ankle joint so your weight shifts onto the balls of your feet; keep your heels down.
2 Lean backward slightly from your ankle joint so your weight shifts onto the heels; the toes should be lengthened and without tension.

3 Place your weight in the centre of each foot, over the arches, and notice a triangle of connection with the floor: points at the base of the big toe, little toe and the centre of the heel. The toes should be active.

4 Lengthen your legs but allow your knees to soften.

5 Tilt your pelvis forward slightly (south, so your pubic bone moves back and your lower back arches a little).

6 Passing through neutral, slightly tilt your pelvis backward (north, so your pubic bone moves forward and your lower back rounds a little).

7 Return your pelvis to neutral, a mid-position where the pubic bone is on same plane as prominent pelvic bones, which are also level with each other.

8 Lengthen your waist equally on both sides.

9 Find your centre by gently recruiting your pelvic floor and deep abdominal muscles (see page 62).

10 Allow your ribcage to relax and be positioned directly above the pelvis, neither swaying backward nor slumping forward.

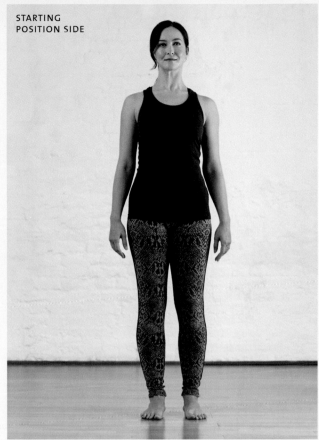

STARTING
POSITION SIDE

STARTING POSITION
FRONT

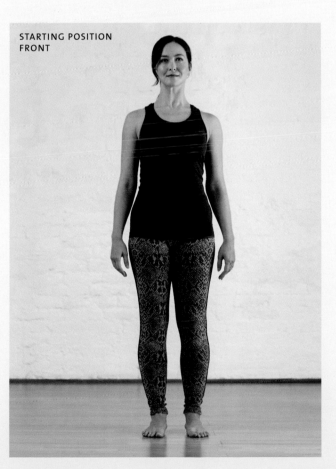

11 Gently lift up through your breastbone.

12 Feel your shoulder blades widen in your upper back, and your collarbones open at the front of your chest. Soften your breastbone.

13 Allow your arms to hang freely in the shoulder sockets. Feel space beneath your armpits and a sense of length and weight through your hands.

14 Release your neck and allow your head to balance freely on top of your spine; sense the crown of your head lengthening up to the ceiling.

15 Relax your jaw muscles and focus your gaze directly forward.

16 While lengthening up, stay grounded through your feet.

17 Breathe naturally into your ribcage.

18 Feel as if you are growing upward dynamically.

PILATES STANCE (LEVEL 1)

This standing position is very useful in helping you "connect" to your deep core. It also subtly helps you engage your deep gluteal and inner thigh muscles. If the inner thighs do not touch, do not force them.

Start standing with your legs slightly turned out from the hips and inner thighs connected.

Connect your heels and turn your toes slightly apart, creating a small V position with the feet.

Relax your arms by the sides of your body.

Follow the Action Points for Standing (see page 58), but connect the entire length of the inner thighs with a sense of drawing them together and up toward the pubic bone.

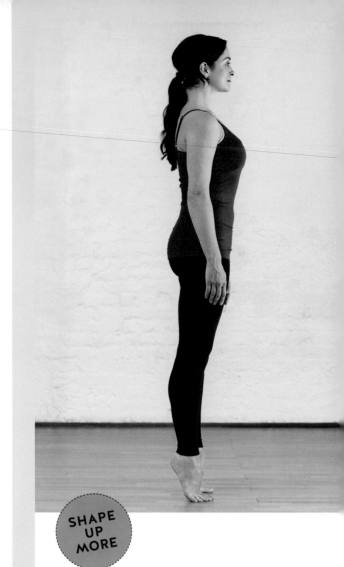

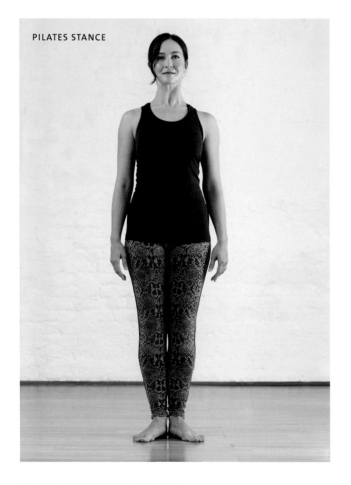

PILATES STANCE

SHAPE UP MORE

Remember these Shape Up More exercises are more challenging. You'll need to master Breathing and Centring before you try them.

Add Heel Raises to Standing and Pilates Stance (Level 2).

To challenge your balance and work your feet and calf muscles, rise onto the balls of your feet as you practise. Ensure that all your toes stay connected with the floor and your ankles and knees do not roll in or out. Then lower the heels but stay tall.

STATIC STANDING LUNGE (LEVEL 4)

This is a relatively new position for Pilates. Joseph Pilates borrowed from lots of other methods and techniques, including yoga, martial arts and ballet. A Lunge is normally dynamic, but for some exercises in the Shape Up programme we use it as a static starting position. You can step forward or backward into the Lunge position. For most people, backward is less challenging. Holding the Lunge position is difficult hence the Level 4 rating (remember to apply the ABCs as you practise). Avoid if you have knee problems.

STARTING POSITION
Stand tall, feet hip-width apart and in parallel.

ACTION

1   Step backward with your right foot, bending the right knee and hip toward 90-degree angles. Your right heel lifts. Simultaneously bend the left knee so the thigh is as near to parallel as you can manage. Stay as upright as possible, challenging your balance and stability.
2   Return to the Starting Position then repeat, stepping back with the left foot.

Once you are confident with this Lunge position, you may step forward into the Lunge.

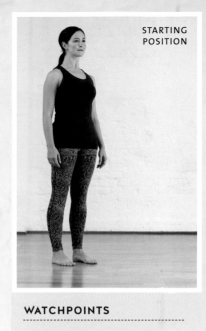

STARTING POSITION

WATCHPOINTS

➔ Use appropriate core connection to control your alignment and movements (see pages 64–65).

➔ Step out only as far as you can maintain good alignment.

➔ Keep your neutral alignment, head, ribcage and pelvis stacked above each other.

➔ Keep your front knee above the ankle and in line with your second toe.

Breathing

*"Therefore, above all, learn
how to breathe correctly."*

JOSEPH PILATES, *RETURN TO LIFE THROUGH CONTROLOGY*

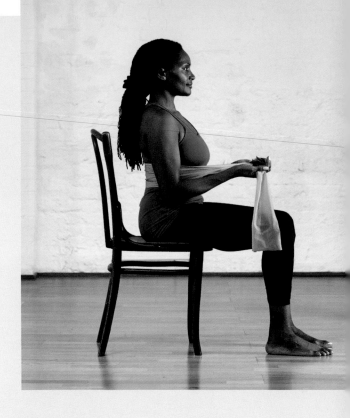

Breathing is an automatic process we rarely think about. Most of us breathe far too shallowly and much faster than we need to, which can limit the supply of oxygen and reduce the ability to eliminate carbon dioxide. If you breathe using mainly the upper part of the chest, you use only a fraction of your lung capacity. If you breathe rapidly, you take a new breath before emptying the lungs of stale air, decreasing your supply of oxygen and thus your energy. Efficient breathing has many health and beauty benefits and encourages good posture. Most exercises in the book use lateral thoracic breathing (Scarf Breathing), a wonderful breathing pattern that helps to mobilize the upper spine.

It's important to think about good alignment before trying a breathing exercise. Efficient breathing relies on good posture, while a hunched position compresses your ribs and thoracic cavity and restricts your main breathing muscle, the diaphragm. In Pilates we focus on a deep, rhythmic way of breathing that encourages the diaphragm to move up and down, which in turn allows the thoracic cavity to expand fully. A full inhalation followed by a deep exhalation increases your capacity to inhale new fresh air.

You can't feel the diaphragm, but it helps to visualize this big dome-shaped muscle separating the thoracic cavity (your ribcage) horizontally from the abdominal cavity. It also helps to visualize the lungs in the ribcage. To help focus on this area, try the following exercise.

SCARF BREATHING (LATERAL THORACIC BREATHING) (LEVEL 1)

The scarf gives sensory feedback to help you feel your ribcage expanding and closing with each breath. Eventually you can practise Scarf Breathing in any of the Starting Positions (see pages 48–60) except Prone, but first we will try it sitting or standing. You will need a scarf or long, light stretch band.

STARTING POSITION
Sit or stand tall and wrap the scarf or stretch band around the lower part of your ribs, crossing it at the front. Hold the opposite ends and gently pull tight.

ACTION: INHALATION
Breathing in through your nose and keeping your shoulders relaxed, focus on the back and sides of the ribcage, where your lungs are located. Feel your lungs expand, like balloons swelling gradually with air, widening the walls of your ribcage. Feel the scarf tightening as your ribs expand. Do not be tempted to force the inhalation – this creates tension.

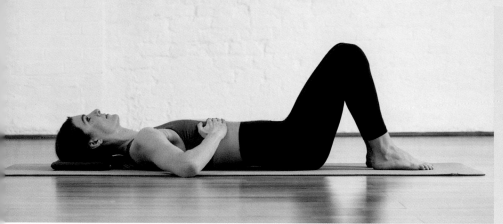

Notice your abdominal area extending outward. Filling the lungs causes the diaphragm to descend into your abdominal area.

ACTION: EXHALATION

As you breathe out, feel the air gently being pushed out fully, as if from the very bottom of your lungs. As your diaphragm begins to rise, feel your ribcage start to close in reaction to your lungs emptying.

TIMING

We use breathing patterns to help facilitate better movement in Pilates practice. However, most people find timing difficult at first, especially if used to other fitness regimes. When you first start practising the exercises, focus on controlling the movements. When those are under control, layer on the breath-control. Most importantly, never hold your breath or force it in any way.

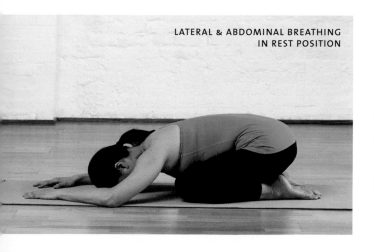

LATERAL & ABDOMINAL BREATHING
IN REST POSITION

THE HUNDRED BREATHING PATTERN (LEVEL 1)

This is a great way to improve your breathing and lung capacity. Full instructions are on page 124. It takes time to master the Hundred pattern of 5 counts for the in-breath, 5 for an out-breath, so start gradually, perhaps breathing in for 3 counts and out for 3 (or 4).

For a relaxing breath rather than an action breath, make your out-breath slightly longer than your in-breath, breathing in for 3 counts and out for 5 for example.

DEEP ABDOMINAL BREATHING FOR RELEASE

We can also use deep abdominal breathing, rather than Pilates' traditional lateral thoracic breathing, to help relax the abdomen and release the pelvic floor. This type of breathing, used frequently in yoga, involves breathing in deeply, allowing your abdomen to fully and completely expand. As you do so, your diaphragm descends and there is a corresponding reaction in the pelvic floor. When practising Pilates you are using your core connection to stay stable (see page 64). To balance this, it's a good idea to do a few deep abdominal breaths before and after your Pilates practice to ensure you are not "holding onto" any tension.

You can practise deep abdominal breathing in different positions. Relaxation Position, Seated in Long Frog and Rest Position are my favourites.

Centring

Here's a Pilates equation for you: A + B = C. If you are in control of your Alignment and your Breathing, you are probably also Centred. By staying in control of what should be moving and what shouldn't, by keeping good alignment of these (moving and non-moving) parts, and by breathing efficiently, you're about there with Centring!

So what do we mean by Centring? The term encompasses many of the popular and widely discussed concepts associated with "stability training". In general terms we say an object is stable if it can cope with the demands placed on it. For example, a stable chair is one built to carry the weight of the person sitting on it, and which also remains upright if knocked. Stability can also be applied to moving objects, for example, a bicycle can be stable or unstable.

In relation to exercise, stability is perhaps best viewed as the ability to maintain control of movements. This may mean stopping undesired movement while allowing desired movements to be performed with maximum efficiency. For example, in a Single Knee Fold (page 69), the pelvis has to be kept still while the leg moves. Whereas in a Spine Curl (page 90), the stability challenge is to move segmentally, bone by bone, through your midline without tipping the pelvis or spine from side to side or hiking up the hip. Every exercise in Pilates has a stability challenge!

Centring, or core stability, is being able to stabilize and control the position of different segments of your body: pelvis, spine, ribcage, shoulders and head. Gaining stability provides a strong and stable, although not necessarily still, base of support from which all Pilates movements are initiated. To do this we have to train the core muscles. Which muscles these are depends on what movement you are doing.

There are many schools of Pilates. Each one has its favourite way to describe how to engage your core muscles. They include cues such as "navel to spine", "use the powerhouse", "stabilize", "zip and hollow" – the list goes on. The words aren't really important, it's the feeling they convey of the connection to inner control. In this section of the book we focus on how to find this connection and use it to control your movements.

Although much of the stability process takes place on a subconscious level, it is possible to train and improve stability throughout the body using conscious control. By practising Pilates we hope to prepare your body to subconsciously react to any demand placed on it by automatically using its deep core muscles. Pilates is based on the principle that by practising control over movements during a session, and repeating good movements, you pattern or ingrain these movements into your mind and body, improving the quality of all movements as you go about your daily activities. Your stability training helps you to develop an inner girdle of strength – a natural in-built corset that wraps around your trunk and supports your spine.

THE DIMMER SWITCH

To remind you about centring, you'll see the following instruction in the exercises:

> ➔ **Use appropriate core connection to control your alignment and movements.**

What do we mean by appropriate? In a class, your teacher would give directions to help you stay stable. Working from a book you have to figure this out for yourself. To help we developed the Dimmer Switch Approach.

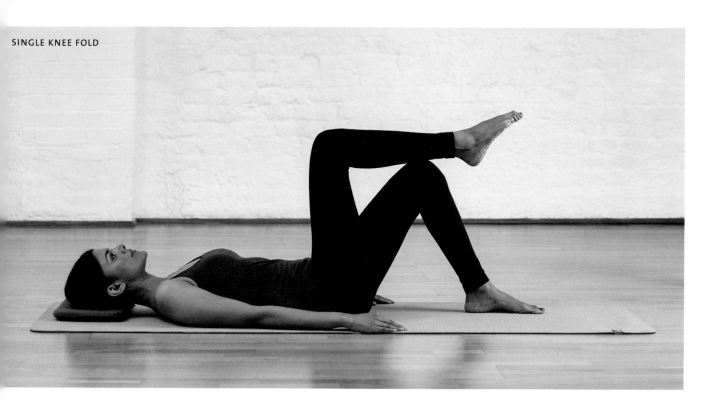

One of the most common mistakes made in Pilates is over-recruiting the core muscles. If you engage these deep muscles too strongly to begin with, you may end up "fixing", becoming rigid or bracing, stifling natural movement. The answer is to only engage your deep core as far as you need to control the movement. No more, no less.

We call this the Dimmer Switch approach – adjusting how strongly you use your core muscles like turning the dial on a dimmer switch up or down. Then you constantly adjust the level to match the demands placed on the body.

The Single and Double Knee Fold (pages 69 and 70) are good examples of how the amount of centring required relates to the challenge of the exercise. You only need to engage your deep muscles gently for the Single Knee Fold, whereas you have to "turn up" the Dimmer Switch and engage your core more strongly as you lift the second leg in the Double Knee Fold.

Once you have mastered connecting to your centre with the exercises on pages 66–67, you can apply what you have learned to all the other exercises in this book. You should eventually become so proficient that you no longer need to actively engage your core – by controlling your alignment through movement it automatically engages.

DOUBLE KNEE FOLD

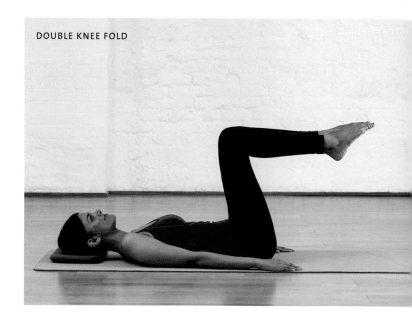

FINDING YOUR CENTRE

WIND ZIP (LEVEL 1)

The focus of this exercise is to feel your deep core muscles and learn how to engage them. As you practise, remember the Dimmer Switch (page 64) and be aware of when to engage these muscles more or less. We are all individuals so, while this varies, your goal remains the same: to stay in control of your alignment and movements.

STARTING POSITION

Sit upright on a chair or your mat. Place your feet on the floor, hip-width apart. Make sure your weight is evenly distributed on both sitting bones and your spine is lengthened in neutral.

Before you engage your core muscles, take a few very deep abdominal breaths right down low into your abdomen. Allow your abdomen to fully expand. This helps you start from a point of "release" before you try to engage.

ACTION

1 Breathe in to prepare, and lengthen through your spine.
2 Breathe out as you gently squeeze your back passage (anus) as if trying to prevent yourself from passing wind. Then bring this feeling forward, toward your pubic bone, as if trying to stop yourself from passing water. Continue to gently draw these pelvic-floor muscles up inside. You should feel your abdominals automatically begin to hollow. Imagine you are engaging an internal zip from back to front and up inside.
3 Maintain this core connection and breathe normally for 5 breaths; your ribs should feel free to move. Then relax completely.

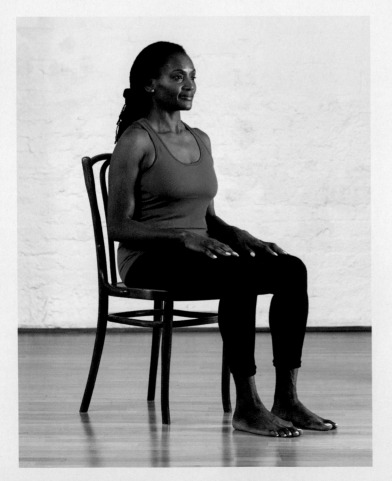

WATCHPOINTS

→ Do not zip, pull up or pull in too hard. It is important not to force this action or to grip.

→ Keep your buttock muscles relaxed and pelvis still.

→ Keep your spine lengthened, your shoulders, face and jaw relaxed.

→ Keep your breathing smooth and evenly paced. If your ribcage and abdominal area expand with your in-breath, this a good sign that you haven't over-engaged.

→ If you lose any of the connections, relax and start again from the beginning.

WATCHPOINTS

➔ When you engage your core muscles do not move your spine or pelvis. That comes later!

➔ Check that you can still breathe easily and that your ribcage is moving.

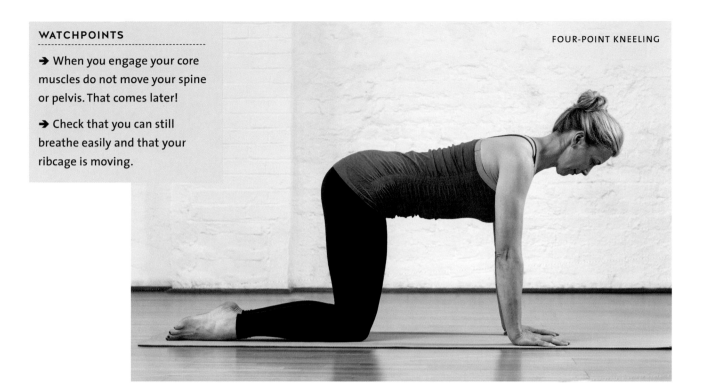

CONNECTING TO YOUR CORE MUSCLES: FOUR-POINT KNEELING (LEVEL 1)

Since we are all individuals, what works for one person may not work for another, so try isolating your core muscles in a variety of positions and ways to find which suits you best.

STARTING POSITION
Four-point Kneeling (page 54).

ACTION

1 Breathe in to prepare.

2 Breathe out as you gently squeeze your back passage (anus) as if trying to prevent yourself from passing wind, then bring this feeling forward, toward your pubic bone. Then draw these muscles up inside until you feel your abdominals automatically begin to hollow.

3 Maintain this connection and breathe normally for 5 breaths before releasing, ensuring that your abdominals and ribs are able to move with your breath.

IDENTIFYING THE PELVIC-FLOOR MUSCLES

Don't worry if you find this difficult – it will become automatic as you practise more.

These tips can help:

· Suck your thumb while drawing up your pelvic floor.

· Alternatively, stick your tongue out!

· Or place your tongue on the roof of your mouth.

· Draw your sitting bones together (this targets the deepest layer of your pelvic-floor).

· Imagine slowing the flow of water as you pass urine.

· For guys, imagine shortening your penis (don't worry, it's not permanent!).

CHALLENGING YOUR CENTRE: CORE STABILITY

Time now to challenge your ability to control the ABCs. In the following exercises, you learn how to move your limbs while keeping the pelvis and spine still. This group of exercises – Leg Slides, Knee Openings, Knee Folds, and Knee Fold and Extend – helps you focus on maintaining a stable relationship between your pelvis and spine, while promoting independent movement of your leg at the hip joint. You can vary which exercises you practise in each session, but the Starting Position is the same for all four. Later in the programme, we will use these exercises again and again to challenge you further.

LEG SLIDES (LEVEL 1)

Initially, you may wish to start by placing your hands on your pelvis to check for unwanted movement. Alternate which leg you start with each time you work out.

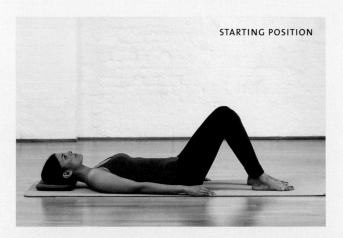

STARTING POSITION

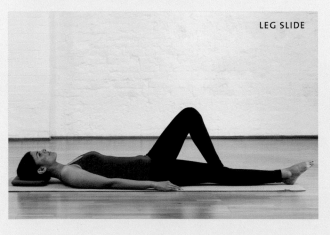

LEG SLIDE

WATCHPOINTS

→ Use appropriate core connection to control your alignment and movements.

→ Keep your pelvis and spine still and centred throughout. Focus on your leg moving in isolation to the rest of your body.

→ Focus on keeping your waist long and even on both sides as you slide your leg in and out.

→ Keep your foot in contact with the floor and in a line with your hip.

→ Keep your chest and the front of your shoulders open, and let go of any tension in the neck area.

STARTING POSITION
Relaxation Position (page 48), arms lengthened alongside you on the mat.

ACTION
1 Breathe in to prepare.
2 Breathe out as you slide one leg away along the floor, in line with your hip. Keep your pelvis and spine stable and in neutral.
3 Breathe in as you draw your leg back in line with your hip to the Starting Position.
4 Repeat 5 times with each leg.

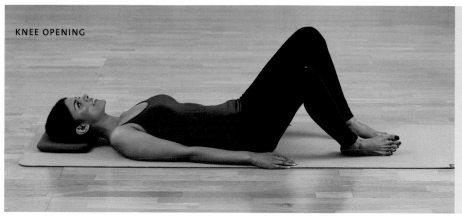

KNEE OPENING

WATCHPOINTS

→ Follow all the Watchpoints for Leg Slides (page 68).

→ Focus especially on not allowing your pelvis to rock to either side.

→ Keep your supporting leg correctly aligned and still; do not allow it to open away from the working leg.

KNEE OPENINGS (LEVEL 1)

STARTING POSITION
Relaxation Position (page 48), arms lengthened alongside you on the mat.

ACTION

1 Breathe in to prepare.
2 Breathe out as you allow one knee to slowly open to the side. Keep the foot on the mat but allow it to roll to its outer border. Open your knee as far as you can without disturbing the neighbours... just checking you were paying attention... the pelvis.
3 Breathe in as you bring the knee back to the Starting Position.
4 Repeat 5 times with each leg.

SINGLE KNEE FOLDS (LEVEL 1)

STARTING POSITION
Relaxation Position (page 48), arms lengthened alongside you on the mat.

ACTION

1 Breathe in to prepare.
2 Breathe out as you lift your right foot off the mat and fold the knee up toward your body. Remain grounded in your pelvis.
3 Breathe in and stay centred.
4 Breathe out as you slowly return the leg down and your foot to the mat.
5 Repeat 5 times with each leg.

WATCHPOINTS

→ Follow all the Watchpoints for Leg Slides (page 68).

→ Do not allow your abdomen to bulge or your pelvis to move. Be especially careful as you begin to lift your leg.

→ Fold your knee in as far as you can without upsetting the pelvis and losing neutral.

→ Fold your knee in directly in line with your hip joint.

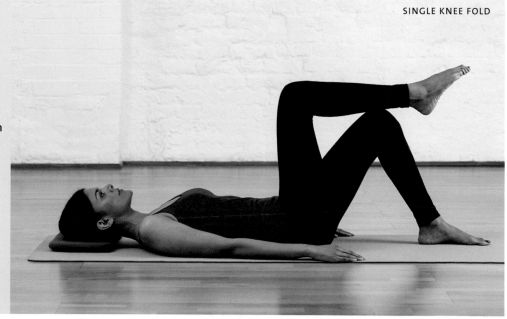

SINGLE KNEE FOLD

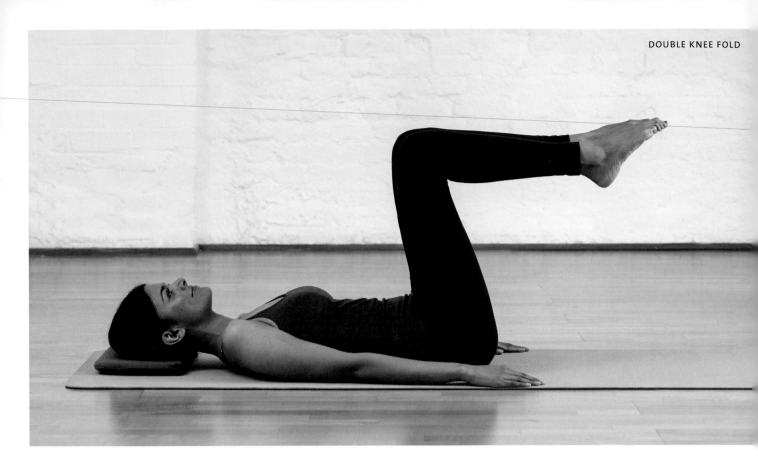

DOUBLE KNEE FOLDS (LEVEL 3)

We've included this exercise here because it forms part of many abdominal exercises in the book. However, it is by no means easy to perform well – don't attempt it until you can confidently practise all the previous exercises in this section. When you can happily do this exercise easily and with control, you may raise and lower each leg, still one at a time, but on a single out-breath.

STARTING POSITION

Relaxation Position (see page 48), arms lengthened alongside you on the mat.

ACTION

1 Breathe in to prepare.
2 Breathe out as you fold your right knee in. Remain grounded in your pelvis and long in your spine.
3 Breathe in; maintain the position and stay centred.
4 Breathe out as you increase your connection to your centre and fold your left knee up and toward you.

5 Breathe in, stay centred, your pelvis remains neutral.
6 Breathe out as you slowly lower your right foot to the mat.
7 Breathe out as you slowly return the left leg down and your foot to the mat.
8 Repeat 6 times, alternating which leg you raise and lower first.

WATCHPOINTS

➔ Use appropriate core connection to control your alignment and movements.

➔ Follow the Watchpoints for Single Knee Folds (page 69).

➔ Remember lifting and lowering your second knee requires much more stability.

➔ Don't forget to breathe.

KNEE FOLD AND EXTEND (LEVEL 2)

We use this leg action repeatedly in the Shape Up programme. It's part of many of Joseph Pilates' original exercises so important to get right.

STARTING POSITION
Relaxation Position (see page 48), arms lengthened alongside you on the mat.

ACTION
Follow Action Points 1 and 2 for Single Knee Fold (page 69), then:

3 Breathe in and maintain the Knee Fold.
4 Breathe out as you straighten your leg to about 45 degrees. Do not disturb your pelvis.
5 Breathe in and fold the knee in.
6 Breathe out and lower the foot to the floor with control.
7 Repeat up to 8 times, alternating legs.

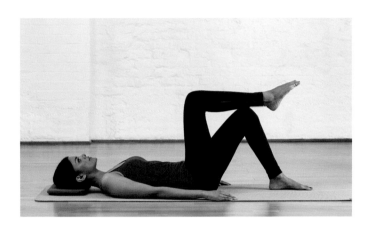

KNEE FOLD & EXTEND

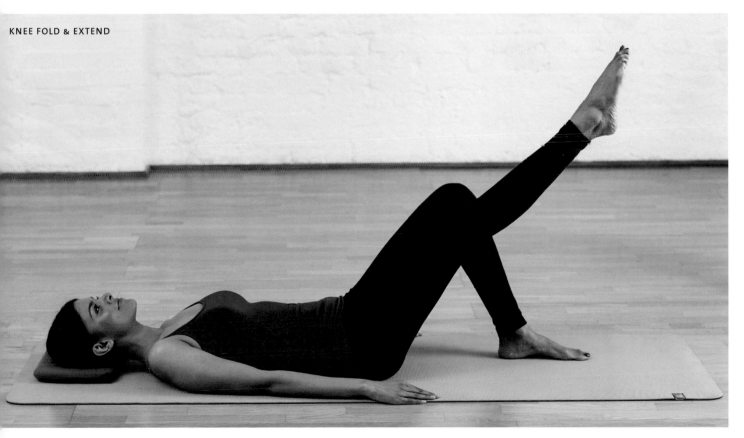

PELVIC STABILITY WITH ARMS UP (LEVEL 3)

We can increase the challenge of all the pelvic stability exercises by lifting the arms up into Shoulder Drop Position (page 78).

Single Knee Fold Arms Up (right)
Leg Slide Arms Up (right)
Knee Fold and Extended Arms (below)
Knee Roll Arms Up (opposite)
Or add an Arm Action e.g Ribcage
Closure (opposite) or Arm Circles
(page 84).

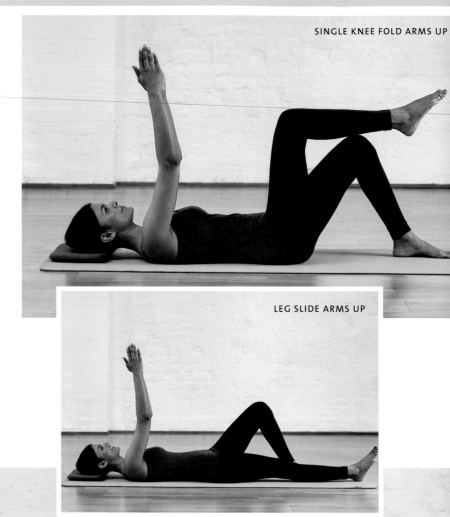

SINGLE KNEE FOLD ARMS UP

LEG SLIDE ARMS UP

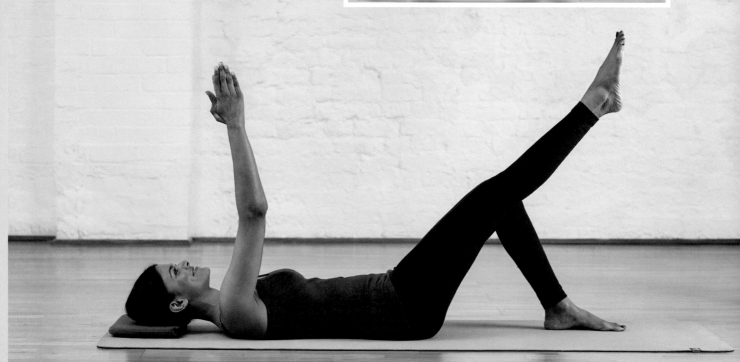

KNEE FOLD & EXTENDED ARMS

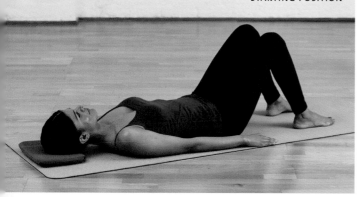

STARTING POSITION

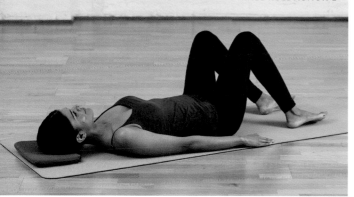

KNEE ROLL ACTION 2

KNEE ROLLS (LEVEL 2)

This exercise mobilizes your hips while challenging your stability, and makes a useful warm-up before a session. We will be adding further challenges to it later.

STARTING POSITION
Relaxation Position (page 48), legs slightly wider than hip-width apart. Reach your arms out to the sides at slightly lower than shoulder-height, palms facing down.

ACTION
1 Breathe in to prepare.
2 Breathe out as you roll your left leg out from the hip joint and simultaneously roll the right leg in, also from the hip joint. Both knees roll to the left. Feet roll too.
3 Breathe in and return both legs to centre at the same time.
4 Breathe out and return both legs to the other side, then repeat the whole sequence up to 5 times.

KNEE ROLLS WITH RIBCAGE CLOSURE ARMS UP 1

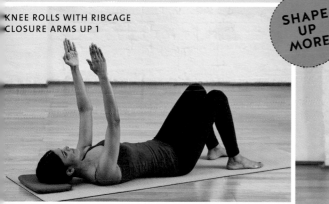

SHAPE UP MORE

KNEE ROLLS WITH RIBCAGE CLOSURE (LEVEL 3)

Start with arms lifted, then take them back as you breathe out and roll your knees. Breathe in to centre the knees and return the arms. Repeat, rolling the knees to the other side.

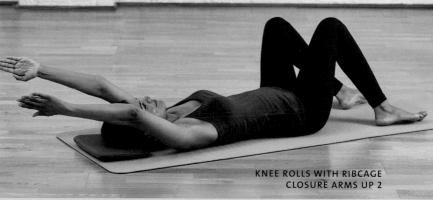

KNEE ROLLS WITH RIBCAGE CLOSURE ARMS UP 2

WATCHPOINTS
- → Use appropriate core connection to control your alignment and movements.
- → Try to keep your pelvis as still as possible.
- → Control the rolling of the knees; don't let them collapse to one side.

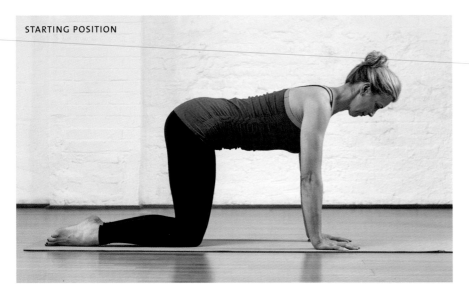

TABLE TOP (LEVEL 2)

Primarily a stability exercise, this also works your arms, shoulders, waist and gluteals. We've broken it down into stages for you to layer up. There are Shape Up More challenges on pages 76 and 77, but don't try them until you have mastered the original.

STARTING POSITION
Four-point Kneeling (page 54).

WATCHPOINTS

➜ Use appropriate core connection to control your alignment and movements.

ACTION: LEVEL 1

1 Breathe in to prepare.
2 Breathe out as you slide one leg behind you, directly in line with your hip. Keep your softly pointed foot in contact with the mat. Do not disturb your pelvis or spine.
3 Breathe in and slide the leg back to the Starting Position.
4 Repeat with the opposite leg.

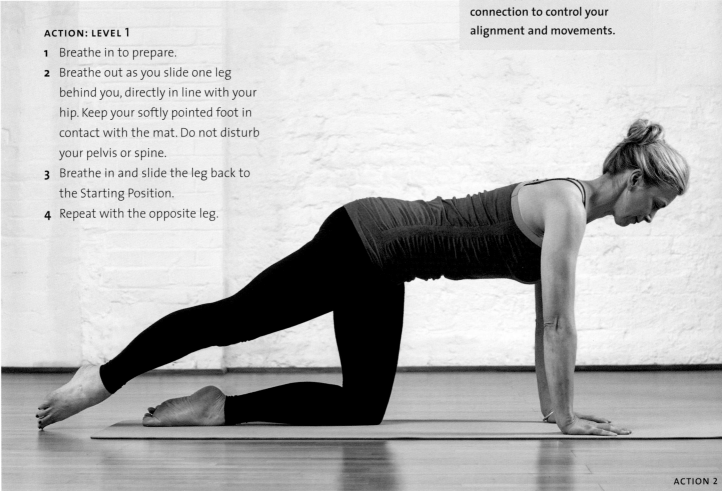

ACTION 2

ACTION: LEVEL 2

Follow Action Points 1–2, then:

3 Breathe in as you lengthen and lift your leg to hip-height, without moving anything else.

4 Breathing out, return the foot to the floor and slide it back in.

5 Repeat with the other leg.

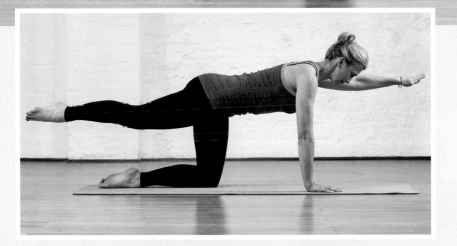

WATCHPOINTS

→ Try to lift your arm to shoulder-height and your leg to hip-height.

→ Keep your pelvis and spine still and neutral throughout.

→ Check that you remain wide and open across your shoulders.

ACTION: LEVEL 3

Follow Action points 1–2, then:

3 Breathe in as you lift the leg to hip-height, simultaneously raising the opposite arm forward, ideally to shoulder-height. Torso stays lengthened and stable.

4 Breathe out and lower your lengthened leg to the mat, simultaneously returning your arm beneath your shoulder.

5 Breathe in and slide your leg back to the Starting Position.

6 Repeat up to 5 times on each side, alternating opposite arm and leg.

TABLE TOP WITH ARM SALUTE (LEVEL 3)

You have to hold good alignment for longer in this version, making it a more challenging exercise.

ACTION

Follow Action Points 1–3, then:

4 As you breathe out, bend your lifted elbow to bring your hand onto your forehead in a salute.
5 Breathe in as you straighten the arm.
6 Breathe out as you return your arms and legs to the Starting Position.
7 Repeat 5 times to each side.

SHAPE UP MORE

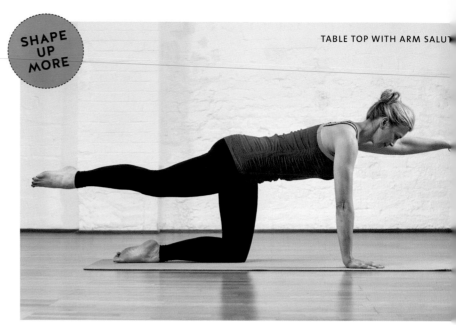

ACTION 4

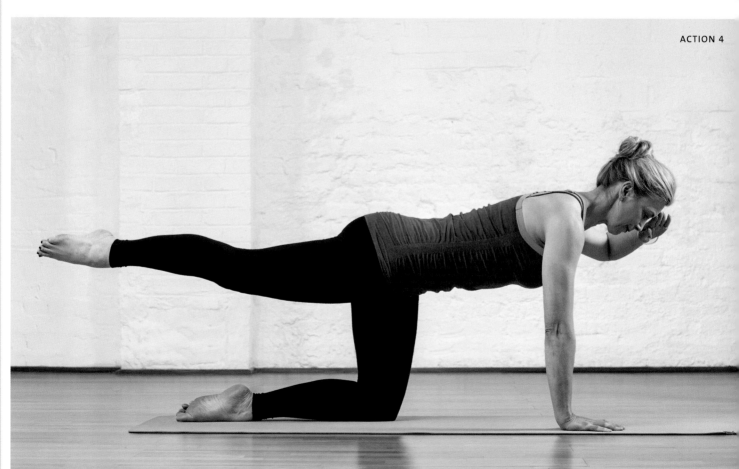

TABLE TOP WITH KNEE BEND (LEVEL 3)

The focus is on the legs now. Practise with or without the opposite arm lifted – of course, a lifted arm provides more challenge.

ACTION
Follow Action Points 1–3, then:

4 Breathe out and bend the lifted knee.
5 Breathe in as you straighten the knee.
6 Breathe out and lower the arm (if using) and leg.
7 Breathe in and return to the Starting Position.
8 Repeat 5 times to each side.

WATCHPOINTS
➜ Use appropriate core connection to control your alignment and movements.

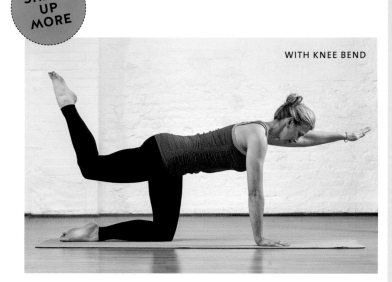

SHAPE UP MORE

WITH KNEE BEND

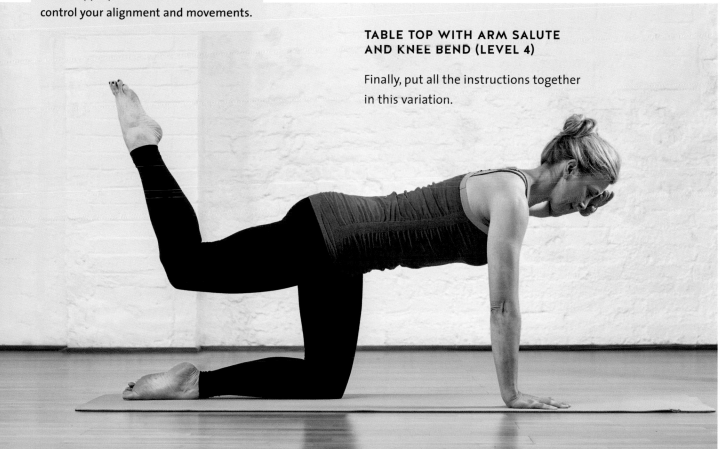

TABLE TOP WITH ARM SALUTE AND KNEE BEND (LEVEL 4)

Finally, put all the instructions together in this variation.

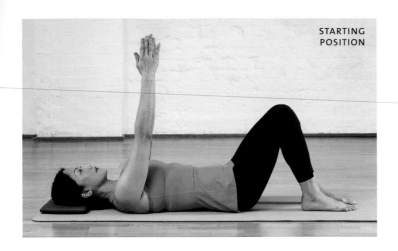

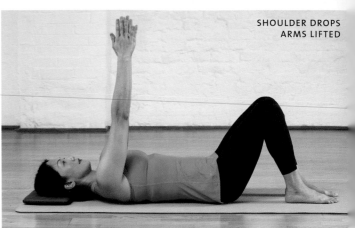

SHOULDER DROPS (LEVEL 1)

So far in the New Fundamentals, (discounting the Shape Up More exercises) we have challenged your core control with the lower limbs. Let's now have a go with the upper limbs. But first we need to get the shoulders organized and in the best place. Shoulder Drops is great for this. This popular exercise releases tension from around the shoulders and neck by mobilizing the shoulder blades. It also helps develop your awareness of how the arms connect to the back of the ribcage via the shoulder girdle. Again, there are Shape Up More options... but master the basic exercise first.

WATCHPOINTS

➜ Keep your pelvis and spine stable and still throughout.

➜ Keep your neck long and free from tension and your head still and heavy throughout.

➜ Fully lengthen your arms, but do not lock your elbows.

STARTING POSITION

Relaxation Position (page 48). Raise both arms vertically above your chest, shoulder-width apart, palms facing one another.

ACTION

1 Breathe in as you reach one arm toward the ceiling, peeling the shoulder blade away from the mat.
2 Breathe out as you gently release the arm back down, returning the shoulder blade to the mat.
3 Repeat up to 10 times, alternating arms.

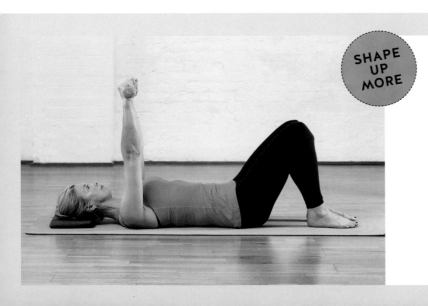

SHAPE UP MORE

DOUBLE SHOULDER DROPS (LEVEL 1)

Reach and release both arms at the same time.

ADD WEIGHTS (LEVEL 2)

Hold light weights in each hand, start with weights up to 0.5kg (1.1lb) for each weight, palms facing away. This adds a toning element but you may also find you get more release using weights.

RIBCAGE CLOSURE (LEVEL 1)

This is a great way to mobilize your shoulders, but your primary goal is to stay in control of the position of your ribcage and upper spine. We combine Ribcage Closure with other exercises later in the book.

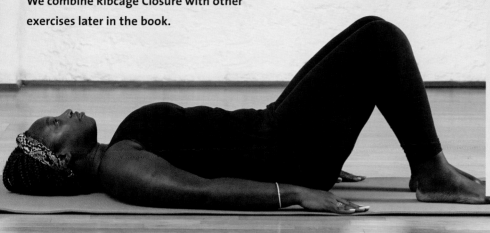

WATCHPOINTS

➜ Use appropriate core connection to control your alignment and movements.

➜ Unless you are very flexible, it is unlikely that your arms will reach the floor behind you. Ear-level is normal.

➜ Be particularly careful not to allow your upper spine to arch as you reach your arms overhead.

➜ Lengthen your arms fully, but do not lock your elbows.

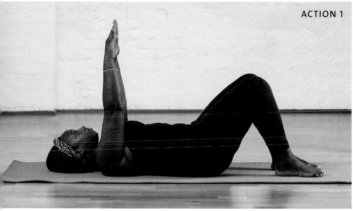

ACTION 1

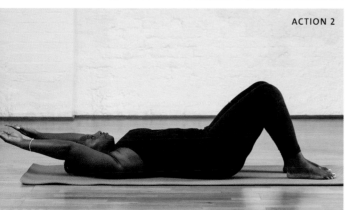

ACTION 2

STARTING POSITION

Relaxation Position (page 48), arms lengthened by your sides, palms facing inward or palms facing down, whichever feels best. Take a moment to notice the weight of your ribs, pelvis and head on the mat – this shouldn't change during the exercise.

ACTION

1 Breathe in and raise both of your arms to shoulder-height.

2 Breath out as you reach both arms overhead, toward the floor. Keep your neck long and encourage your ribcage to soften and close, with your spine still and stable.

3 Breathe in as you return the arms above your chest. Feel your ribcage heavy and your collarbones opening.

4 Breathe out and lower the arms, lengthening as you return them to your sides.

5 Repeat up to 10 times.

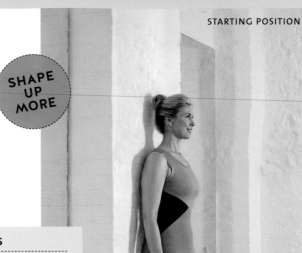

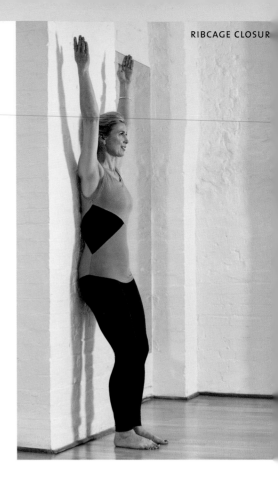

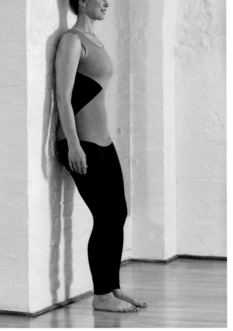

SHAPE UP MORE

WATCHPOINTS

→ Use appropriate core connection to control your alignment and movements.

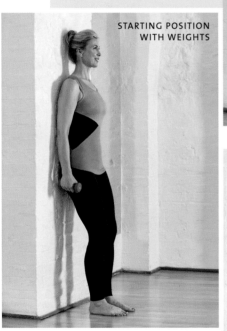

STARTING POSITION WITH WEIGHTS

RIBCAGE CLOSURE AGAINST A WALL (LEVEL 2)

Stand about 30cm (1ft) from a wall, then sit back into the wall, feet hip-width apart and parallel. Bend your knees softy to help your alignment, checking it against the wall. Be aware of the back of your head, ribcage and pelvis against the wall, and your spine retaining its natural curves. The back of your head may not touch the wall. This is fine; don't tip it back, just lengthen up through the crown of the head. Then follow the directions for lying Ribcage Closure (page 79), substituting the wall for the floor.

RIBCAGE CLOSURE AGAINST A WALL WITH WEIGHTS (LEVEL 3)

Practise holding light weights in each hand – initially no more than 0.5kg (1.1lb) each.

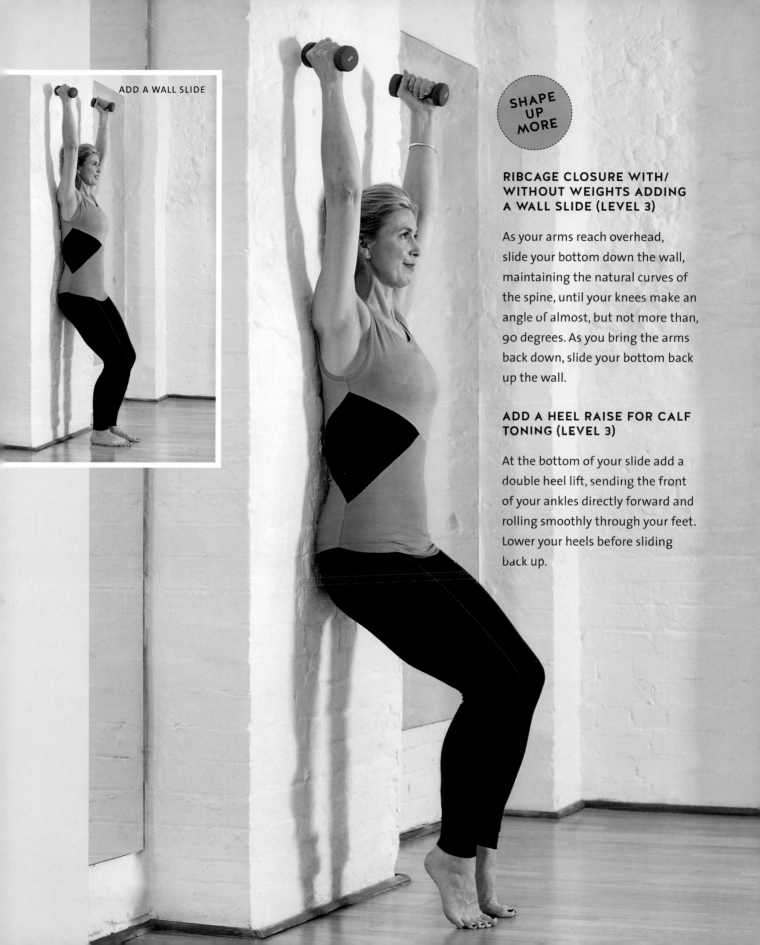

ADD A WALL SLIDE

SHAPE UP MORE

RIBCAGE CLOSURE WITH/ WITHOUT WEIGHTS ADDING A WALL SLIDE (LEVEL 3)

As your arms reach overhead, slide your bottom down the wall, maintaining the natural curves of the spine, until your knees make an angle of almost, but not more than, 90 degrees. As you bring the arms back down, slide your bottom back up the wall.

ADD A HEEL RAISE FOR CALF TONING (LEVEL 3)

At the bottom of your slide add a double heel lift, sending the front of your ankles directly forward and rolling smoothly through your feet. Lower your heels before sliding back up.

SINGLE FLOATING ARMS (LEVEL 1)

This action features a lot in the standing exercises. The movement skills you learn here can be used whenever you need to raise your arms in an exercise. Many of us overuse the upper part of our shoulders – it's why these muscles can get really tense. This simple exercise helps you find a way of lifting the arms that doesn't overuse these muscles.

STARTING POSITION

Stand tall in Parallel (page 58) or Pilates Stance (page 70) – you could also use High Kneeling (page 57), Seated positions (page 53) or Static Standing Lunge (page 61). Place your right hand on your left shoulder. Feel your collarbone: try to keep it still in the first part of the movement, your hand checking that the upper part of the shoulder remains "quiet" for as long as possible.

ACTION

1 Breathe in to prepare.
2 Breathe out as you slowly begin to raise one arm, reaching wide out of the shoulder blades like a bird's wing. Think of your little finger leading the arm, with the arm following the hand as it floats outward. Keep your arm just in front of your shoulders, within your peripheral vision. Allow the arm to rotate naturally within the shoulder socket as it lifts.
3 Breathe in as you lower the arm to your side, following the same pathway.
4 Repeat 3 times with each arm.

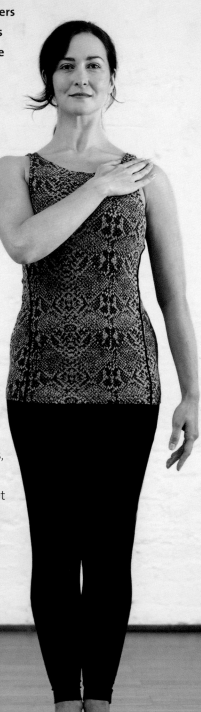

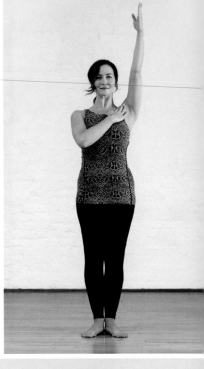

WATCHPOINTS

➔ Use appropriate core connection to control your alignment and movements.

➔ As you raise your arm, think of this order of movement: arm, shoulder blade, collarbone.

➔ Allow the shoulder blade to glide.

➔ Add an extra breath, if you need to.

➔ Do not allow your upper body to shift to the side; stay centred.

➔ Maintain the distance between ear and shoulder.

DOUBLE FLOATING ARMS (LEVEL 1)

Simply float both arms up simultaneously.

DOUBLE FLOATING ARMS WITH WEIGHTS (LEVEL 2)

Use light weights, initially no more than 0.5kg (1.1lb) each. For a change, as the arms return down, turn the palms to face downward. This gives a wonderful sense of growing up through the crown of the head – think swan rather than duck.

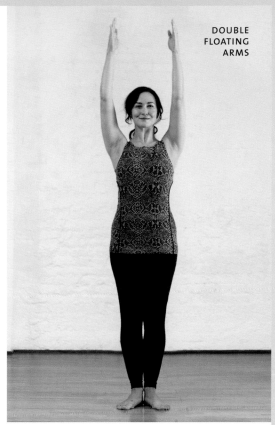

DOUBLE FLOATING ARMS

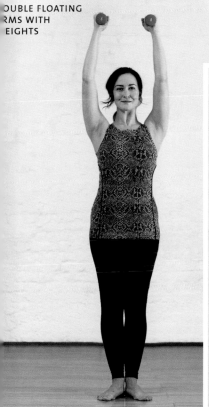

DOUBLE FLOATING ARMS WITH WEIGHTS

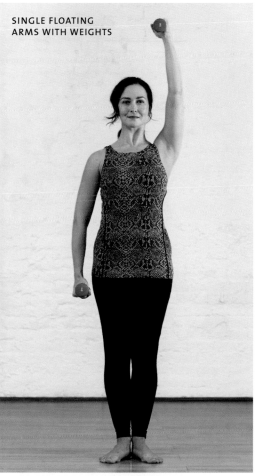

SINGLE FLOATING ARMS WITH WEIGHTS

SINGLE FLOATING ARMS WITH WEIGHTS (LEVEL 3)

Stand for this version. With only one arm working and the added weight, you have to work harder to stay centred and balanced (it's easier to float both arms up simultaneously). Resist the temptation to lean to one side.

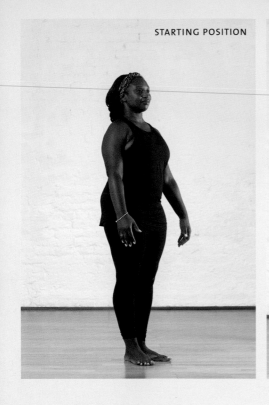

STARTING POSITION

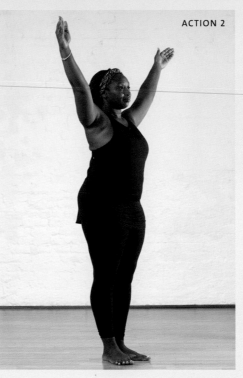

ACTION 2

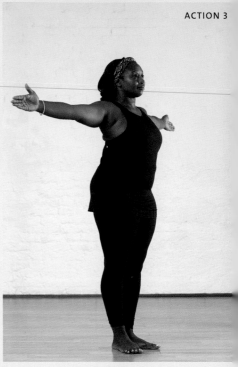

ACTION 3

ACTION 4

WATCHPOINTS

➔ Use appropriate core connection to control your alignment and movements.

➔ Enjoy the free movement of your arms and shoulders but try to keep your ribcage connected down toward your waist and your upper spine still.

➔ Remember what you learned in Floating Arms (page 82): the arm moves first, then as the arms reach overhead, allow the shoulder blades to glide smoothly around the ribcage.

➔ As the arms circle, keep them on the same level as each other.

ARM CIRCLES (LEVEL 2)

This exercise mobilizes your shoulders and feels great whichever starting position you choose.

STARTING POSITION
Relaxation Position (page 48), Standing in Parallel (page 58), Pilates Stance (page 60), High Kneeling (page 56), High Kneeling Lunge (page 56) or Static Standing Lunge (page 61). You can add these circles to many different exercises, such as Standing Back Bends (page 184).

ACTION
1   Breathe in to prepare.
2   Breathe out as you raise both arms overhead, without disturbing your spine, ribcage or pelvis.
3   Breathe in as you circle your arms out to the side and take them slightly behind you (if in an upright position) before you return the arms to the starting positiony.
4   Once your arms are below shoulder-height you may take them slightly behind you before you return the arms to the starting position.
5   Repeat 5 times, then reverse the direction.

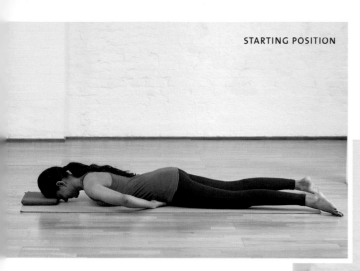

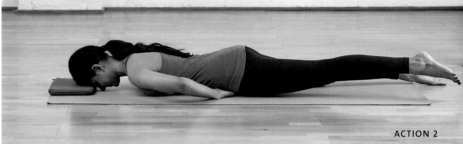

ACTION 2

WATCHPOINTS

→ Keep your core connected to support your lower back.

→ Raise your leg only as high as you can without disturbing your pelvis and spine.

→ Fully lengthen your legs but do not lock your knees.

STAR PREP (LEVEL 1)

This is not just a great stability exercise, it's also good for toning the gluteal muscles of your buttocks.

STARTING POSITION

Prone (page 58) with a folded towel or flat cushion beneath your forehead. Place your fingertips just under your pelvic bones. Your legs are straight, slightly wider than hip-width apart and turned out from the hips, or have the legs in parallel. Note the pressure (or lack of pressure) on your fingertips. Your goal is not to increase or decrease this pressure – not as easy as it sounds.

ACTION

1 Breathe in to prepare.
2 Breathe out as you lengthen and lift one leg off the mat without disturbing the pelvis or spine. You should not feel any change to the pressure on your fingertips.
3 Breathe in as you lengthen and lower your leg back down to the mat.
4 Repeat up to 10 times, lifting alternate legs.

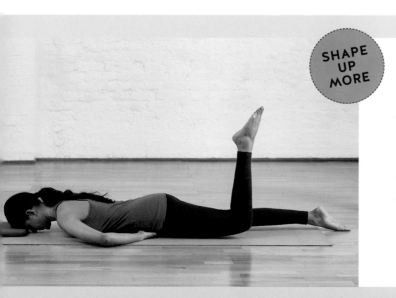

SHAPE UP MORE

STAR PREP KNEE LIFTS (LEVEL 3)

To isolate the gluteal muscles even more, and increase the strengthening effect, start with legs in parallel and hip-width apart. Follow all the directions with a bent knee, lengthening the knee away from your hip.

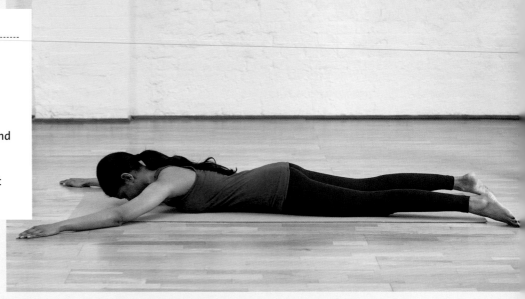

WATCHPOINTS

➔ Use appropriate core connection to control your alignment and movements.

➔ Lift your leg only as high as you can maintain a still and stable pelvis and spine.

➔ Keep your arms down but your spine lifted.

HALF STAR (LEVEL 4)

Great for your back, shoulder and buttock muscles.

STARTING POSITION
As for Star Prep but with arms reaching above you and resting on the mat, slightly wider than shoulder-width, palms down.

ACTION
1 Breathe in to prepare.
2 Breathe out as you sequentially lift your head, neck and upper spine into a Diamond Press (page 106) position, ribs staying down. Shine your breastbone forward and up.
3 Breathe in and lengthen through the spine.
4 Breathe out as you lengthen and lift one leg slightly off the mat without disturbing your spine or pelvis.
5 Breathe in as you lower your leg back to the mat.
6 Repeat up to 10 times before lengthening back down to the Starting Position.

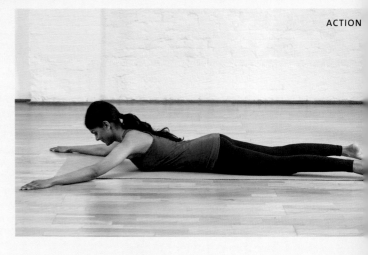

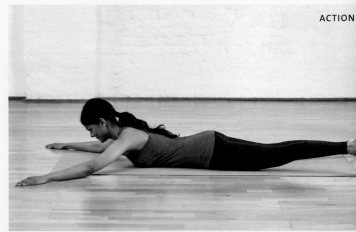

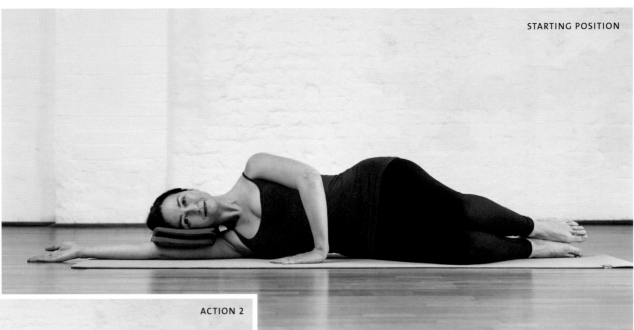

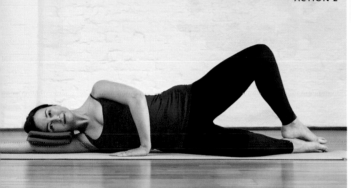

ACTION 2

WATCHPOINTS

→ Use appropriate core connection to control your alignment and movements.

→ Stay aligned, shoulder above shoulder, hip above hip, knee above knee.

→ Move your top leg only as far as you can without disturbing the position of your pelvis and spine.

→ Keep lengthening both sides of the waist throughout.

→ The top arm is positioned to help support you, but don't place too much weight on it.

→ Keep your chest open and your focus directly ahead.

OYSTER (LEVEL 1)

Use this exercise to isolate and tone the gluteal muscles.

STARTING POSITION

Lie on your right side, in a straight line, stacking your shoulders, hips and ankles. Lengthen your right arm beneath your head and in line with your spine: you will probably need a flat cushion or folded towel to keep your head in line with your spine. Place your left hand in front of your ribcage. Bend both knees, feet drawn back so your heels align with the back of your pelvis.

ACTION

1 Breathe in to prepare.
2 Breathe out as you open your top knee, keeping your feet connected. This "turn out" movement comes from your hip joint. Keep your pelvis still and stable.
3 Breathe in and, with control, return your leg to the Starting Position.
4 Repeat up to 10 times, then repeat on the other side.

VARIATION: You may place a pillow between your knees if you wish.

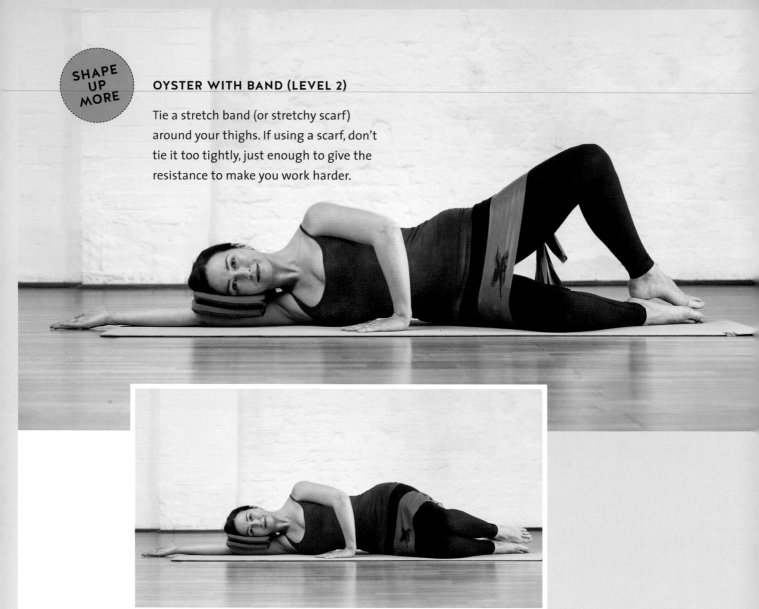

OYSTER WITH BAND (LEVEL 2)

Tie a stretch band (or stretchy scarf) around your thighs. If using a scarf, don't tie it too tightly, just enough to give the resistance to make you work harder.

SIDE-LYING KNEE CROSS OVERS WITH ARMS UP (LEVEL 4)

Tougher still, have your top arm above you to make your core work harder and challenge your balance.

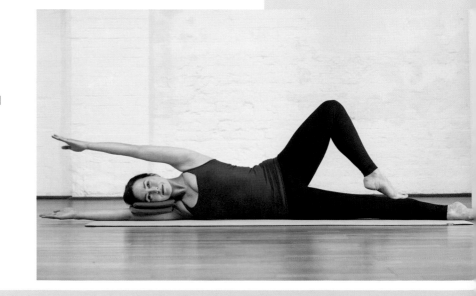

SHAPE
UP
MORE

SIDE-LYING KNEE CROSS OVERS (LEVEL 3)

This version of Oyster adds an element of balance and takes the hip through a wider range of movement. Start with your underneath leg straightened in line with your body and your top working leg bent, foot resting on the lower calf.

Follow the Oyster Action Points but allow the knee to roll forward, inwardly rotating the thigh bone in the hip socket. Don't let your pelvis roll forward.

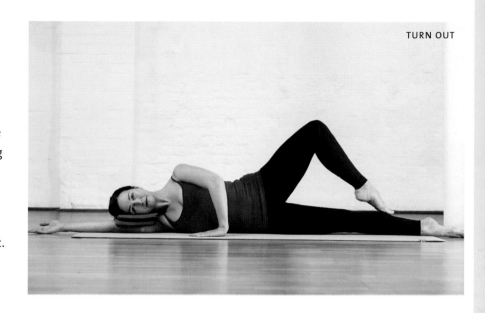

TURN OUT

TURN IN

WATCHPOINTS

→ Use appropriate core connection to control your alignment and movements.

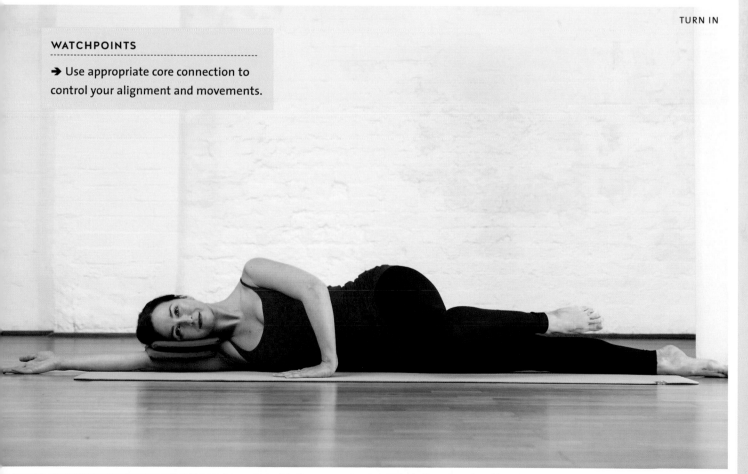

MOBILITY

So far in the programme, we've asked you to move your limbs while keeping your pelvis and spine still. It's now time to challenge your stability through movement. A balanced workout includes all the movements the spine can make: flexion, rotation, side flexion and extension.

SPINE CURLS (LEVEL 1)

Everyone's favourite, this exercise teaches you how to articulate the spine (move it bone by bone) and also works the gluteals and abdominals. The Shape Up More versions of this exercise are much more challenging. Do wait until you are ready before trying them – you need to be very stable to do them successfully.

WATCHPOINTS

➔ Use appropriate core connection to control your alignment and movements.

➔ Take equal weight through both feet. This helps to prevent your pelvis from dipping to either side.

➔ Lengthen the waist equally on both sides.

➔ Keep the knees parallel, in line with your hips, and don't let your feet roll in or out.

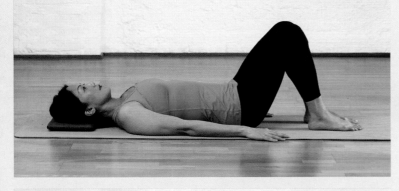

STARTING POSITION

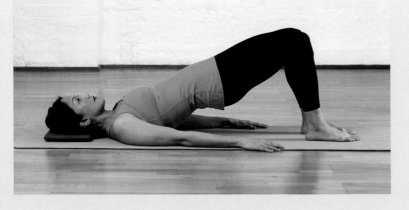

ACTION 3

STARTING POSITION
Relaxation Position (page 48), arms lengthened by the side of your body.

ACTION
1 Breathe in to prepare.
2 Breathe out as you curl your tailbone under, tilting the pelvis to north, then peel your spine off the mat one vertebra at a time, lengthening your knees away from your hips. Roll your spine sequentially, bone by bone, up to the tips of the shoulder blades.
3 Breathe in and hold this position, focusing on the length in your spine.
4 Breathe out as you roll the spine back down, softening the breastbone and wheeling each bone down in turn.
5 Breathe in as you release the pelvis back to level.
6 Repeat up to 10 times.

ADD A KNEE OPENING

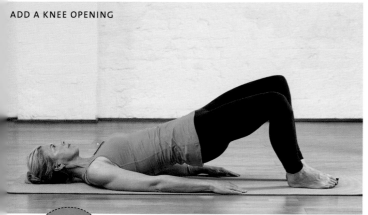

ADD A KNEE FOLD

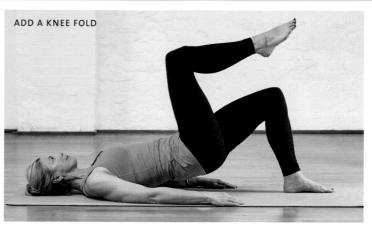

SHAPE UP MORE

ARMS UP

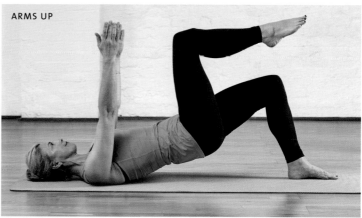

ADD A KNEE OPENING (LEVEL 3)

At the top of the Spine Curl, check you have lengthened into neutral, then take one knee to the side as in Knee Openings (page 69). Return the knee to centre before rolling down.

ADD A KNEE FOLD (LEVEL 4)

Up the challenge even more to work one buttock really hard. Don't let your pelvis dip to one side. You will probably need to turn up your Dimmer Switch and use more core.

ARMS UP (LEVEL 5)

With your arms raised for Knee Folds, you can make it even tougher.

ADD A RIBCAGE CLOSURE OR ARM CIRCLE (LEVEL 3)

Start with arms by your side, take them back at the height of the Spine Curl, then return your arms to your side before rolling back down. Your challenge is to keep the ribcage connection as the arms go back.

AND THEN… ADD A HEEL RAISE (LEVEL 5)

ADD A RIBCAGE CLOSURE OR ARM CIRCLE

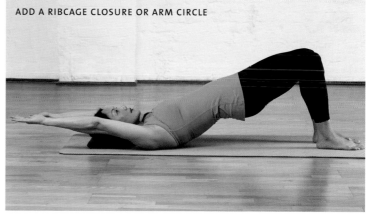

ADD A HEEL RAISE

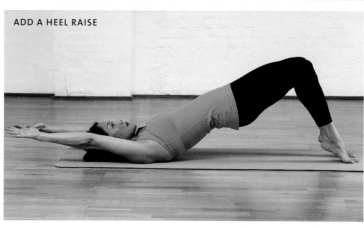

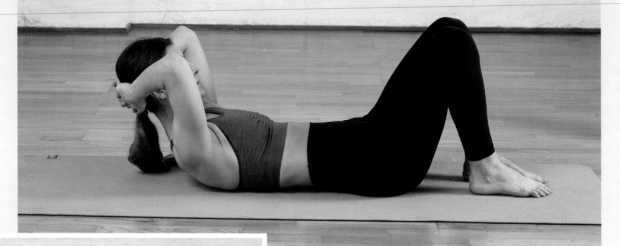

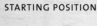
STARTING POSITION

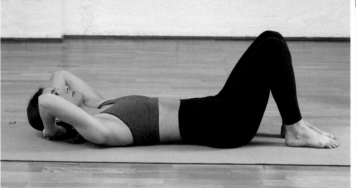

CURL UPS (LEVEL 1)

Done properly, with control, this flexion exercise is one of best abdominal exercises ever. But pay close attention to the detail please or you'll miss out.

STARTING POSITION

Relaxation Position (page 48). Lightly clasp both hands behind your head, keeping your elbows open and positioned just in front of your ears, within your peripheral vision.

ACTION

1 Breathe in to prepare.
2 Breathe out as you lengthen the back of your neck, nod your head and sequentially curl up the upper body, keeping the back of your lower ribcage in contact with the mat. Keep your pelvis still and level and do not allow your abdominals to bulge.
3 Breathe in to the back of your ribcage and maintain the curled-up position.
4 Breathe out as you slowly and sequentially roll the spine back down to the mat with control.
5 Repeat up to 10 times.

WATCHPOINTS

➔ Use appropriate core connection to control your alignment and movements.

➔ Make sure that the pelvis remains in neutral throughout.

➔ Your head stays supported by your hands.

➔ Focus on wheeling your spine off the mat vertebra by vertebra.

➔ Add an extra breath to curl higher, if you wish.

After mastering Curl Ups, challenge yourself by adding a Knee Opening (page 69), a Knee Fold (page 69) or a Leg Slide (page 68). Then progress to the other variations, each adds its own challenge.

You may decide to Curl Up first then, with an extra breath, add a Knee Opening, Knee Fold etc. Or, and this is harder, Curl Up and simultaneously Leg Slide, Knee Fold etc. If you move simultaneously the difficulty goes up to Level 4.

KNEE OPENING (LEVEL 3)

Breathe in as the knee opens, out as it closes.

LEG SLIDE (LEVEL 2)

Slide the leg on the in breath, return on the out breath. Keep the leg in line with the hip.

SINGLE KNEE FOLDS (LEVEL 3)

As before, use the in breath to fold up and the out breath to replace the foot.

DOUBLE KNEE FOLD (LEVEL 4)

Adjust the breathing pattern according to what works best for you.

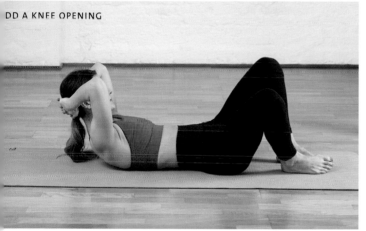

DD A KNEE OPENING

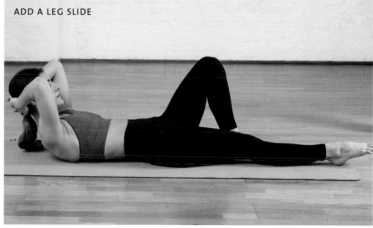

ADD A LEG SLIDE

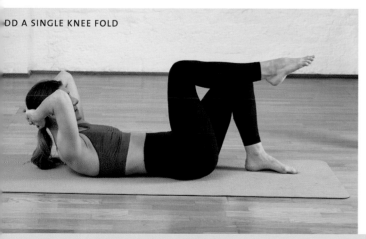

DD A SINGLE KNEE FOLD

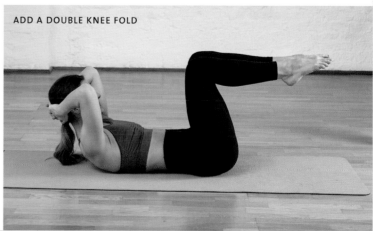

ADD A DOUBLE KNEE FOLD

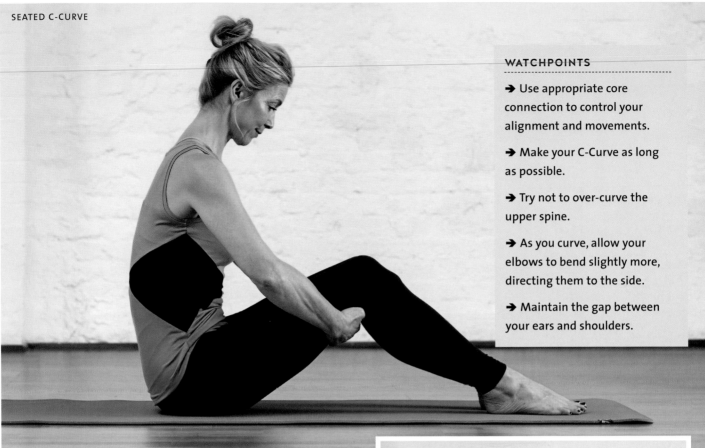

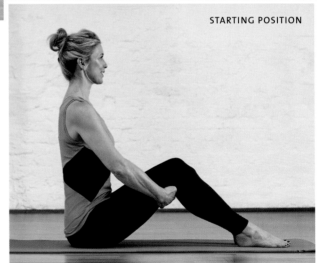

STARTING POSITION

SEATED C-CURVE (LEVEL 2)

Don't expect to get this exercise perfect first time – it is hard and takes practice. But do persevere because it is used a lot later in the programme. A mirror is helpful to check you've arrived in the correct position.

STARTING POSITION
Sit tall, knees bent, soles of your feet on the mat and legs hip-width apart. Place your hands behind your thighs with elbows slightly bent and wide.

ACTION

1 Breathe in as you roll your pelvis back by curling your lower spine underneath you. At the same time, curl your head, neck and upper back forward, creating a lengthened and equally curved spine. Your shoulders should remain vertical over your hips.

2 Breathe out and, moving the pelvis and head simultaneously, lengthen your spine back to neutral.

3 Repeat up to 5 times.

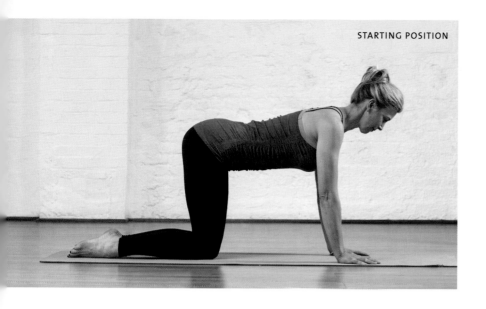

→ Use appropriate core connection to control your alignment and movements.

→ Aim for an elongated C-Curve evenly flexed throughout the spine. A common mistake is to overly round the upper back.

→ Keep your head following the curved line of your spine; do not drop it too far.

→ Keep the weight evenly distributed between both hands and both knees.

→ Fully lengthen your arms but do not lock your elbows.

CAT (LEVEL 1)

This is a great way to keep your spine flexible. First you use the C-Curve in this exercise and then we take you into a gentle back extension.

STARTING POSITION
Four-point Kneeling Position (page 54).

ACTION
1 Breathe in to prepare.
2 Breathe out as you roll your pelvis underneath you, as if directing your tailbone between your legs. As you do so, your lower back gently rounds and then your upper back, followed by your neck. Finally, nod your head slightly forward.
3 Breathe in wide.

4 Breathe out as you simultaneously start to unravel the spine, sending the tailbone away from the crown of your head, and return to neutral.
5 Breathe in and hold your lengthened spine.
6 Breathing out, gently start to extend your upper spine, lengthening first through your head and neck, then shining your breastbone forward. The collarbones are wide and open.
7 Breathe in and return to neutral.
8 Repeat up to 8 times.

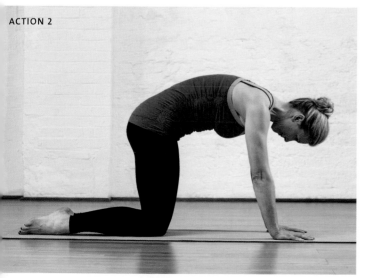

ACTION 2

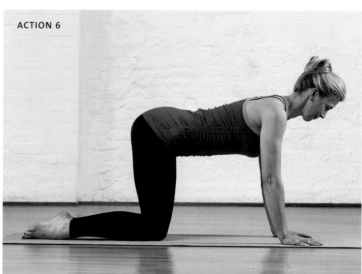

ACTION 6

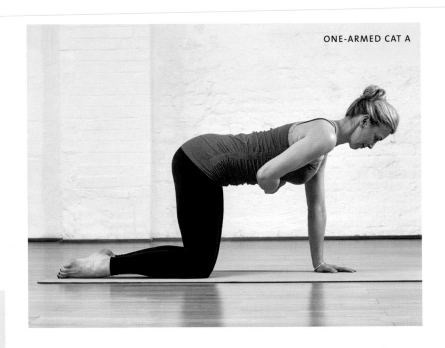

ONE-ARMED CAT A

ONE-ARMED CAT (LEVEL 3)

Start in Three-Point Kneeling (page 55)
and follow Action Points 1–4 (page 95).
The difficulty is to move the spine as
centrally as you can. This works your
arms and shoulders while challenging
your core. You may not achieve much
back extension with this version, which
is why we stop at Action Point 4.

WATCHPOINTS

➔ Use appropriate core
connection to control your
alignment and movements.

ONE-ARMED CAT B

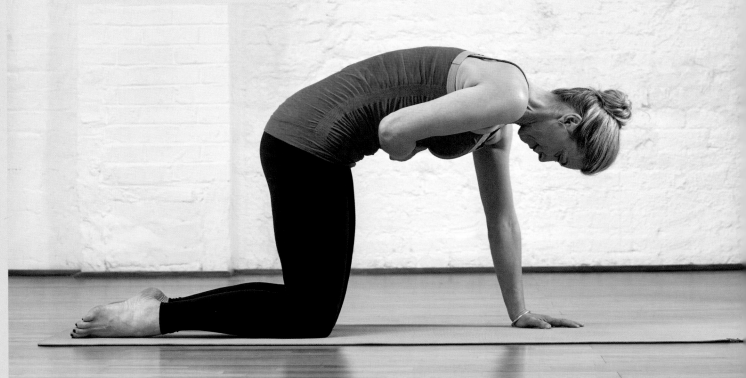

WAIST TWIST (LEVEL 1)

Spinal rotation now. The muscles that help you twist are the same ones that define your waist. As with all our exercises, lengthen up through the crown of the head, spiralling up, up, up as you move into the exercise and on returning to the Starting Position. This spinal rotation will be combined with other movements later in the programme.

STARTING POSITION

Standing in Parallel (page 58), Pilates Stance (page 60), Seated Long Frog (page 53), High Kneeling (page 56) or Lunge positions (page 61).

Sit, stand or kneel tall. If standing or kneeling have the legs parallel and hip-width apart. Fold your arms in front of your chest, just below shoulder-height. Place one palm on top of the opposite elbow and position the other beneath the opposite elbow.

ACTION

1 Breathe in and lengthen up through your spine.
2 Breathe out as you move first your gaze to the right, then turn your head and neck and finally rotate your torso fully to the right. Keep your pelvis still and keep lengthening up through the crown of the head.
3 Breathe in as you continue to lengthen your spine and rotate back to the Starting Position.
4 Repeat 6 times to each side. After 3 turns, change arm position so the bottom arm is on top.

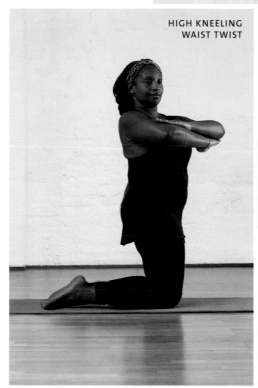

HIGH KNEELING
WAIST TWIST

STANDING STARTING
POSITION

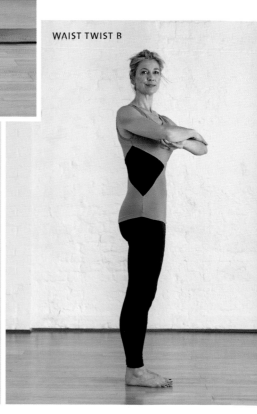

WAIST TWIST B

WATCHPOINTS

➔ Use appropriate core connection to control your alignment and movements.

➔ Your pelvis remains still.

➔ Keep your weight even on both feet (both sitting bones if seated, both knees if kneeling).

➔ Avoid arching your back or shortening your waist.

➔ Carry your arms with your spine; do not allow them to lead.

WAIST TWIST IN HIGH
KNEELING STARTING
POSITION

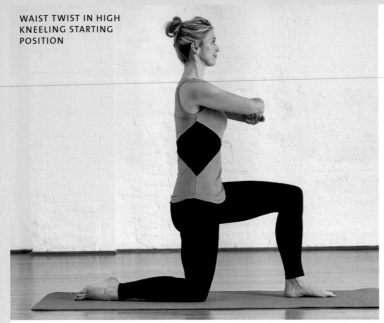

WAIST TWIST IN HIGH
KNEELING LUNGE 2

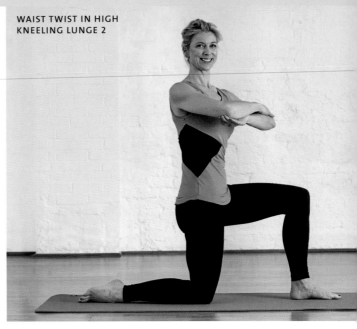

WAIST TWIST IN STATIC
STANDING LUNGE 1

SHAPE
UP
MORE

WAIST TWIST IN HIGH KNEELING LUNGE (LEVEL 3)

By doing Waist Twist in a High Kneeling
Lunge you also work on your balance and
core. Twist both ways. You may wobble.

WAIST TWIST IN STATIC STANDING LUNGE (LEVEL 4)

Twist both ways, then repeat with the
other leg forward.

WAIST TWIST IN STATIC
STANDING LUNGE 2

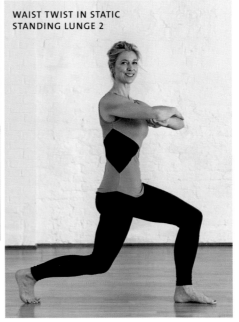

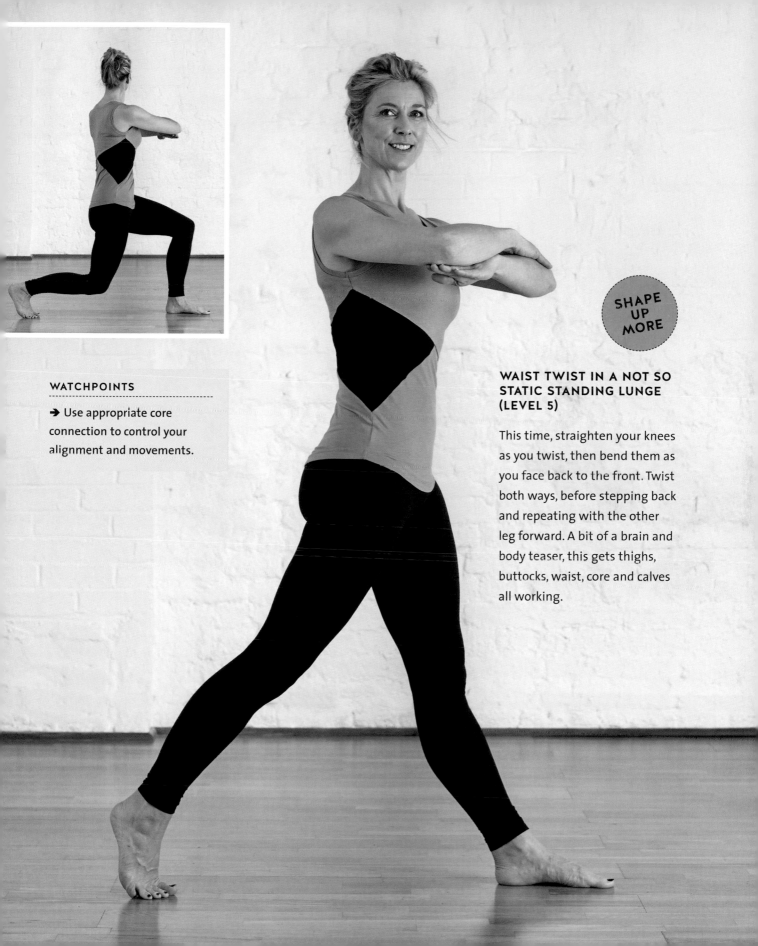

WATCHPOINTS

→ Use appropriate core connection to control your alignment and movements.

WAIST TWIST IN A NOT SO STATIC STANDING LUNGE (LEVEL 5)

This time, straighten your knees as you twist, then bend them as you face back to the front. Twist both ways, before stepping back and repeating with the other leg forward. A bit of a brain and body teaser, this gets thighs, buttocks, waist, core and calves all working.

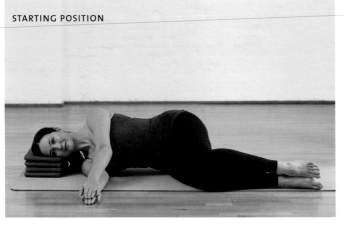

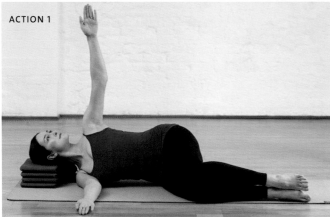

ACTION 1

ARM OPENINGS (LEVEL 1)

A fantastic feel-good exercise that subtly works your waist.

STARTING POSITION

Side-lying Chair Position (page 57), with a pillow or cushion beneath your head to keep your head in line with your neck and spine. Bend both knees in front of you so your hips and knees are at a right angle. Lengthen both arms in front of your body at shoulder-height. Rest one hand on the other.

ACTION

1 Breathe in as you raise the top arm, keeping it straight and lifting it above the shoulder joint toward the ceiling. Simultaneously roll your head and neck to face the ceiling.
2 Breathe out as you continue to rotate your head, neck and upper spine, carrying your arm with you. Keep your pelvis still.
3 Breathe in as you start to rotate back, bringing the arm halfway to above the shoulder.
4 Breathe out as you return to Starting Position.
5 Repeat up to 5 times, then repeat on the other side.

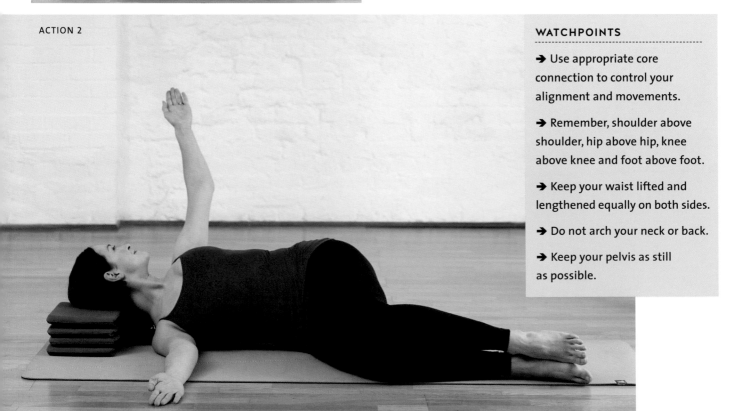

ACTION 2

WATCHPOINTS

→ Use appropriate core connection to control your alignment and movements.

→ Remember, shoulder above shoulder, hip above hip, knee above knee and foot above foot.

→ Keep your waist lifted and lengthened equally on both sides.

→ Do not arch your neck or back.

→ Keep your pelvis as still as possible.

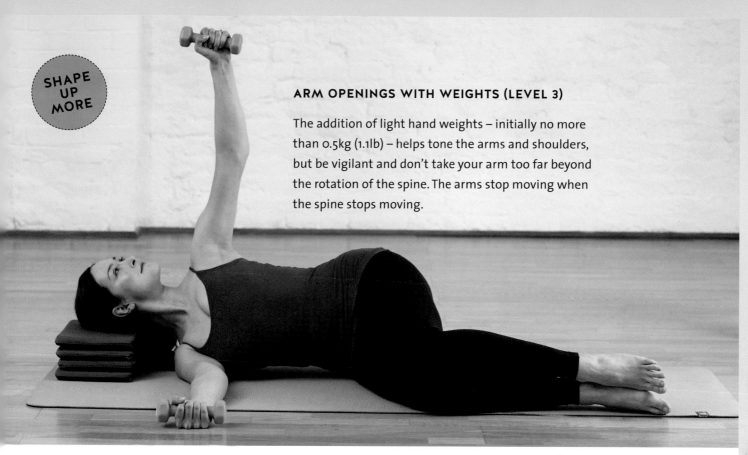

ARM OPENINGS WITH WEIGHTS (LEVEL 3)

The addition of light hand weights – initially no more than 0.5kg (1.1lb) – helps tone the arms and shoulders, but be vigilant and don't take your arm too far beyond the rotation of the spine. The arms stop moving when the spine stops moving.

BUTTERFLIES (LEVEL 2)

This version doesn't add toning power but is useful if you don't have a pillow to hand. Start with hands lightly clasped behind your head so your head rests on your hands. Then open your top elbow as you breathe in, and breathe out to rotate first the head, then the neck, upper spine and finally allow the ribs to rotate around. Return in reverse order.

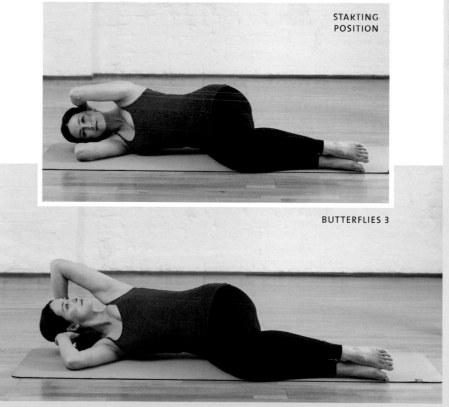

STARTING POSITION

BUTTERFLIES 3

HIP ROLLS (LEVEL 1)

The goal here is to challenge your ability to control the sequential rotation of your spine. It also helps to trim your waist.

STARTING POSITION

Relaxation Position (page 48). Bring your legs together and connect your inner thighs. Reach your arms out on the mat slightly lower than shoulder-height, palms facing upward.

ACTION

1 Breathe in to prepare.
2 Breathe out as roll your pelvis to the left – like rolling west in the Compass (page 50). The right side of your pelvis and lower right ribs peel off the mat slightly.
3 Breathe in as you return the pelvis and legs to the Starting Position, initiating from your centre.
4 Repeat to the other side, then repeat the sequence up to 5 times.

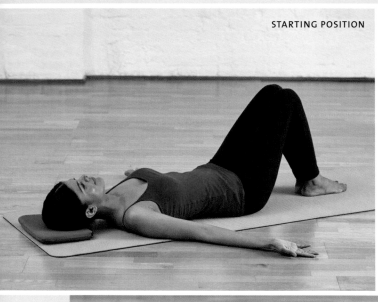

STARTING POSITION

WATCHPOINTS

→ Use appropriate core connection to control your alignment and movements.

→ Roll your pelvis and legs directly to the side; avoid any detours.

→ Keep both sides of your waist equally long.

→ Roll first through your hips, waist and finally your lower ribs.

→ Return first your lower ribs, waist and finally your hips.

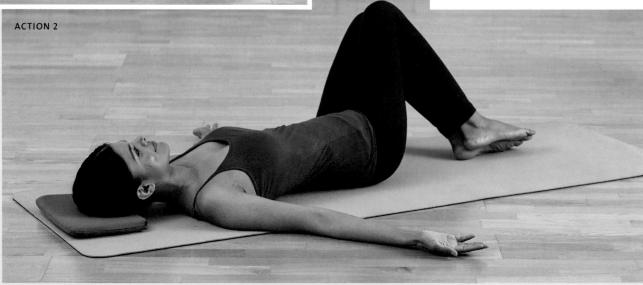

ACTION 2

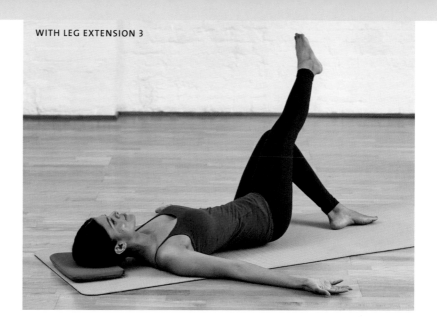

HIP ROLLS WITH LEG EXTENSION (LEVEL 3)

Now add extra challenge to your core by straightening a leg. This increases the load and makes your waist muscles work harder!

Follow Action Points 1 and 2, then:

3 Breathe in and straighten your right leg, keeping the inner thighs glued together.
4 Breathe out as you roll back with control in reverse order: ribs, waist, then hips returning to centre.
5 Breathe in and bend the knee.
6 Repeat 5 times to each side.

HIP ROLLS WITH RIBCAGE CLOSURE (LEVEL 4)

This combination exercise really stretches out your waist while working it. The key is to stay in control of your mid-section. Start with both arms above your shoulders, palms facing each other. Take the arms behind you in a Ribcage Closure (page 79) as you do the Hip Roll, returning them to the Starting Position as your knees return. Do not reach too far back with the arms.

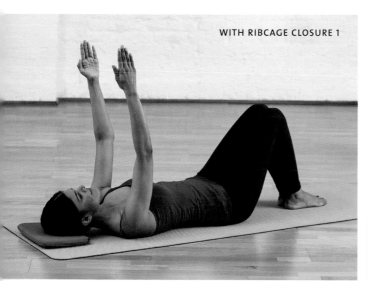

WITH RIBCAGE CLOSURE 1

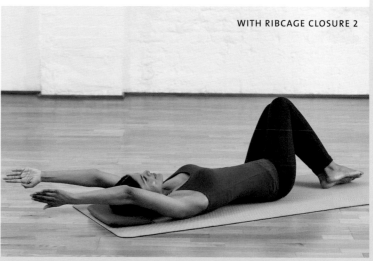

WITH RIBCAGE CLOSURE 2

STARTING POSITION

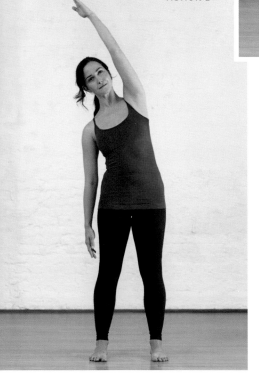

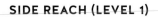

SIDE REACH (LEVEL 1)

If you're looking for a great way to trim down, this feel-good exercise doesn't just stretch your waist, it also tones it.

ACTION 1

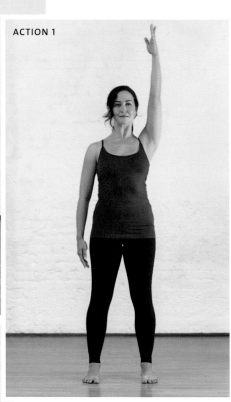

STARTING POSITION

Standing in Parallel (page 58) or Pilates Stance (page 60), Seated Long Frog (page 53), High Kneeling (page 56), High Kneeling Lunge (page 56), Static Standing Lunge (page 61).

If standing, stand tall on the floor (not your mat), legs parallel and shoulder rather than hip-width apart. Lengthen your spine and lengthen your arms by your sides.

ACTION

1 Breathe in as you raise your left arm out to the side and overhead.

2 Breathe out as you reach up and over, leading with your head and sequentially bending your spine to the right.

3 Breathing in, keep lengthening up and focus on breathing laterally.

4 Breathe out as you return your spine to the vertical position. Lower your left arm by your side.

5 Repeat 5 times to each side.

ACTION 2

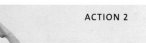

WATCHPOINTS

→ Use appropriate core connection to control your alignment and movements.

→ Move in one plane only, without curving forward or arching back.

→ Keep your head and neck in line with your spine.

→ Keep your weight even on both feet if standing, both sitting bones if seated, and both knees if high kneeling.

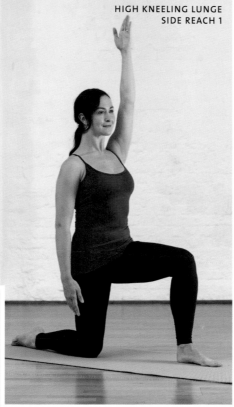

HIGH KNEELING LUNGE
SIDE REACH 1

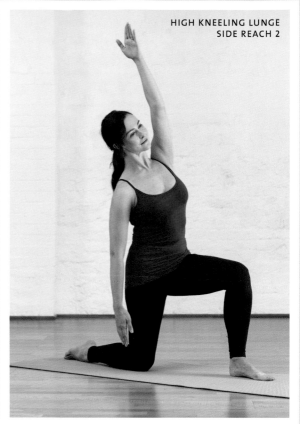

HIGH KNEELING LUNGE
SIDE REACH 2

TATIC STANDING
UNGE SIDE REACH 1

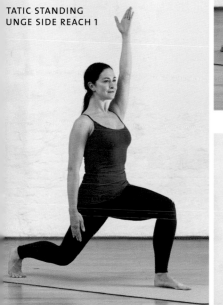

STATIC STANDING LUNGE
SIDE REACH 2

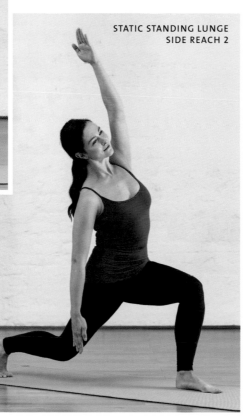

HIGH KNEELING LUNGE SIDE REACH (LEVEL 4)

Changing Starting Position makes a huge difference to the level of difficulty, adding balance and coordination challenges into the mix to make you work your core more. Reach both ways 3 times, then repeat with the other leg forward.

STATIC STANDING LUNGE SIDE REACH (LEVEL 4)

Reach both ways 3 times again, and repeat with the other leg forward to get the thighs, buttocks, waist, core and calves all working harder. You are welcome!

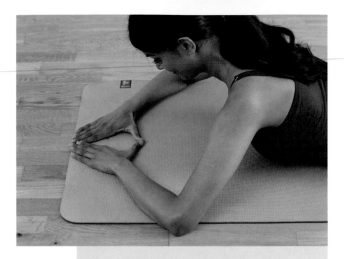

DIAMOND PRESS (LEVEL 1)

We tend to forget about our backs – we look in
the mirror front and side, but rarely check out the
rear view. If you practise these back-extension
exercises, your upper back will be toned and your
posture perfect from every angle.

STARTING POSITION

Prone (page 58), with legs hip-width apart and parallel.
Create a diamond shape with your arms, placing the
fingertips of both hands together, palms on the mat.

Open your elbows. Rest your forehead on the backs of the
hands (or a towel). Place a folded towel or flat cushion under
your abdomen to support your lumbar spine, if wished.

If it is more comfortable you may widen your hand position.

WATCHPOINTS

→ Use appropriate core connection to
control your alignment and movements.

→ Grow, grow, grow forward...

→ Lift your head first (think of rolling
a marble away along the mat with your
nose) and then your neck. When your
head and neck are in line with your spine,
start to extend the upper spine.

→ Keep your lower ribs in contact with
the mat as you lift; this ensures you don't
lift too far and compress your lower spine.
Length is more important than height.

→ Keep your feet in contact with the
mat throughout.

→ As you return to the mat, do not
collapse; return with length and control.

STARTING POSITION

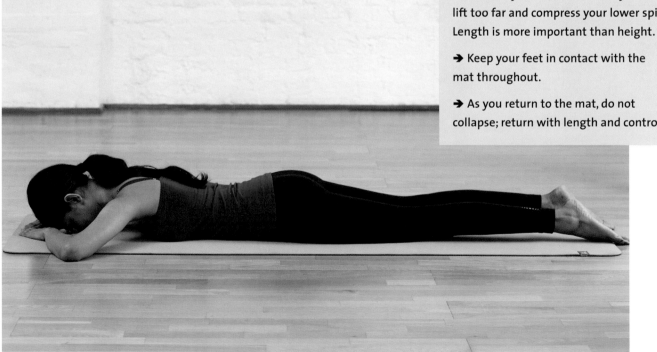

ACTION

1 Breathe in to prepare.

2 Breathe out as you lift first your head, then your neck and finally your chest off the mat. Feel your lower ribs in contact with the mat but shine your breastbone forward, opening your chest.

3 Breathe in as you hold this lengthened position.

4 Breathe out as you lengthen and return your chest, neck and head back to the Starting Position.

5 Repeat up to 10 times.

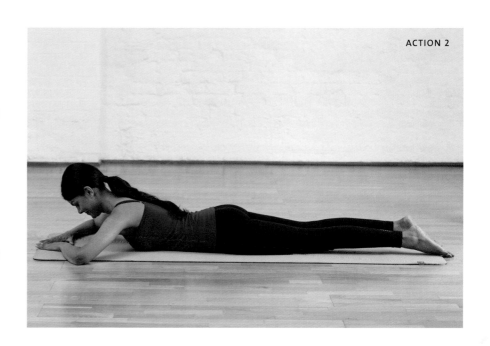

ACTION 2

DIAMOND PRESS SALUTE

SHAPE UP MORE

DIAMOND PRESS SALUTE WITH LEG LIFT (LEVEL 4)

As you salute, lengthen and lift the opposite leg as in Star Prep (page 85). This adds some buttock toning. Repeat 5 times with each arm and leg before returning to the Starling Position.

DIAMOND PRESS SALUTE (LEVEL 3)

Your back muscles have to work harder as you salute in this variation.

Follow Action Points 1 and 2, then:

3 Breathe in and salute your hand to your forehead.

4 Breathe out and return the hand.

5 Repeat 4 times with each hand, then sequentially curl the spine back down.

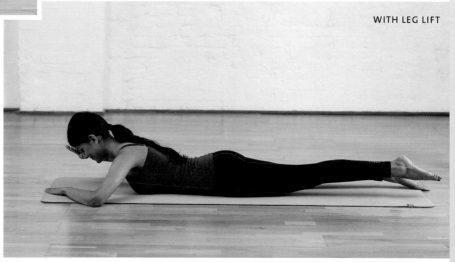

WITH LEG LIFT

REST POSITION (LEVEL 1)

**Use this position after any prone or Four-point Kneeling exercises (page 54).
It is also a great way to encourage either lateral breathing (page 62), or Deep
Abdominal Breathing (page 63). Both provide an opportunity to re-focus
concentration in preparation for the next exercise. You'll find Rest Position
in most of the workouts at the back of the book (pages 197–218).**

STARTING POSITION

From a prone position come up into
Four-point Kneeling (page 54).

ACTION

1 Breathe in and lengthening
   your spine, bring your feet slightly
   closer together.
2 Breathe out as you begin to fold
   at the hips, and direct your buttocks
   backward and down.
3 Keep your hands on the mat and
   lengthen your arms. Try to rest your
   sitting bones on your heels, chest on
   your thighs and forehead on the mat.
4 Breathe in and direct the breath into
   the back and sides of your ribs; feel
   the ribcage progressively expand.

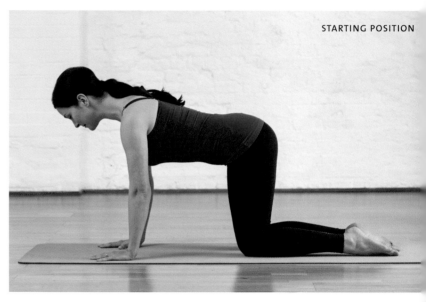

STARTING POSITION

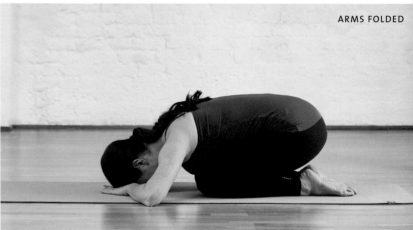

ARMS FOLDED

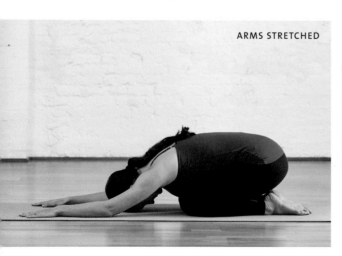

ARMS STRETCHED

5 Breathe out, fully emptying your lungs, and focus on
   closing the ribs down and together. Repeat up to 10 times.
6 To finish, breathe out and begin rolling your pelvis
   underneath you, then sequentially roll and restack your
   spine to an upright position, sitting back on your heels.

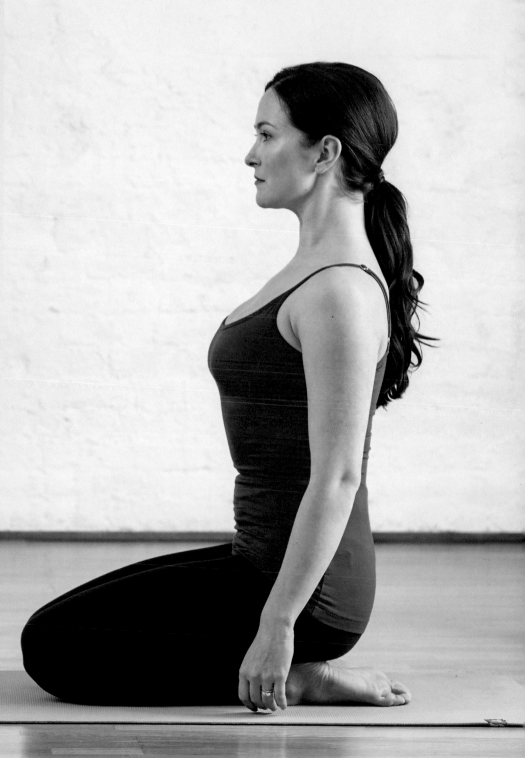

WATCHPOINTS

➔ Use appropriate core connection to control your alignment and movements.

➔ Don't open your knees too wide; the thighs should be slightly apart and beneath the ribcage.

➔ Allow your head to be heavy and your neck lengthened and relaxed.

➔ Depending on your flexibility, you may need to rest your head on cushions (or your folded hands) and/or you may need cushions beneath your bottom.

ROLL DOWNS

Although not really a New Fundamental exercise, Roll Downs are very useful and the perfect way to finish a session.

ROLL DOWNS AGAINST A WALL (LEVEL 2)

Use these Roll Downs to mobilize your spine and hips and encourage support from the abdominals as you strengthen the muscles of your back, buttocks and legs.

STARTING POSITION

Stand tall with your back against a wall. Have your feet parallel, hip-width apart 30–60cm (1–2ft) from the wall, bending your knees slightly. Check your spine retains its natural curves, your pelvis is neutral. The back of your head may or may not be in contact with the wall depending on your posture. Allow your arms to lengthen by the sides of your body.

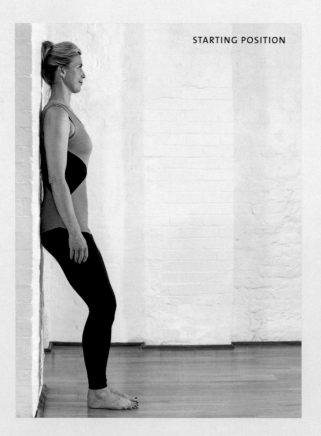

STARTING POSITION

WATCHPOINTS

➔ Roll smoothly and sequentially through each segment of the spine.

➔ Use your deep core connection to support your spine.

➔ As you roll down, begin the movement with a nod of your head.

➔ As you roll up, begin the movement by rolling your pelvis underneath.

➔ Roll directly through your centre-line, avoiding any deviation to either side.

➔ Keep your weight balanced evenly on both feet.

➔ Do not allow your feet to roll either in or out – this is especially important if you rise onto your toes (see page 112).

ACTION

1 Breathe in as you lengthen the back of your neck and nod your head forward.
2 Breathe out as you continue to roll the whole of your spine forward and down. Peel each vertebra from the wall in turn, until you can wheel no more, then bend forward from the hips.
3 Breathe in wide.
4 Breathe out as you roll your pelvis under and restack the vertebrae, rolling the spine back up the wall.
5 Repeat up to 5 times.

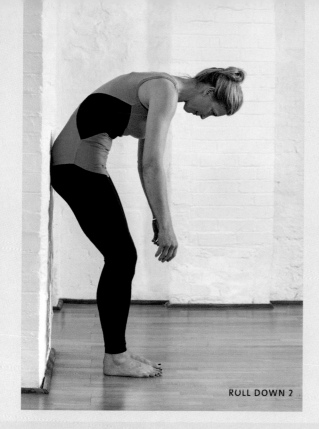

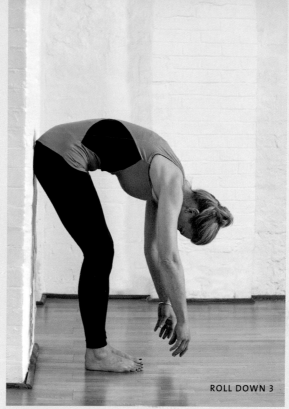

ROLL DOWN 2

ROLL DOWN 3

SHAPE UP MORE

FREE-STANDING ROLL DOWNS (LEVEL 3)

To make the exercise harder, step away from the wall.
Keep your knees softly bent.

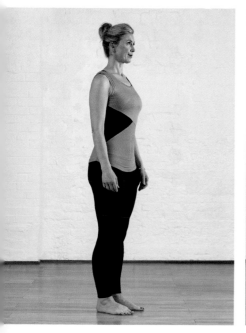

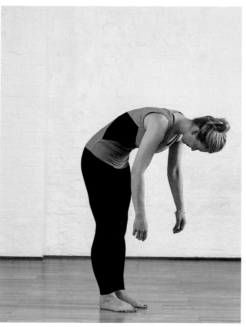

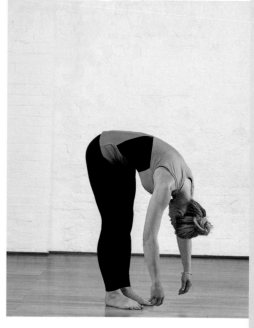

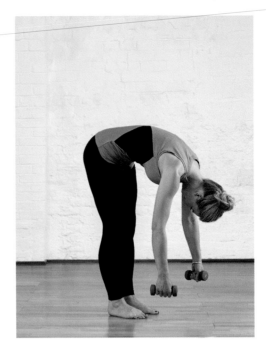

ROLL DOWNS
WITH WEIGHTS

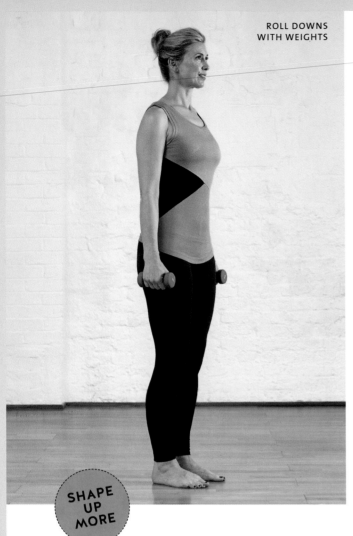

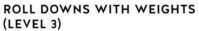

ADD A HEEL RAISE

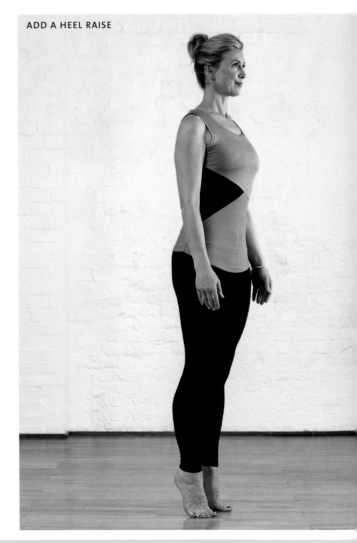

**SHAPE
UP
MORE**

ROLL DOWNS WITH WEIGHTS
(LEVEL 3)

Holding weights – no more than
0.5kg (1.1lb) – does not add much in
terms of extra toning, but it does
feel good.

ROLL DOWNS AND HEEL RAISE
(LEVEL 4)

Once you've rolled back up to
Standing, rise up onto the balls
of your feet. Lower the heels before
rolling down again. Raising the
heels adds toning for the calves
and challenges your balance.

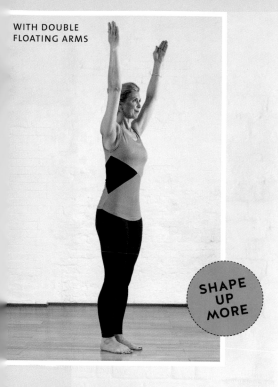

WITH DOUBLE
FLOATING ARMS

SHAPE
UP
MORE

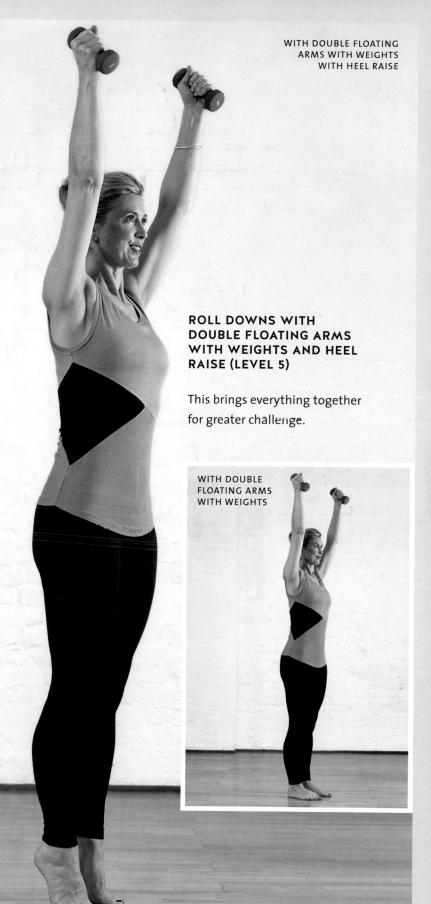

WITH DOUBLE FLOATING
ARMS WITH WEIGHTS
WITH HEEL RAISE

WITH DOUBLE
FLOATING ARMS
WITH WEIGHTS

ROLL DOWNS WITH DOUBLE FLOATING ARMS (LEVEL 3)

Roll down, restack the spine to stand tall, then pause a moment to take an extra breath before floating both arms up. Lower the arms before rolling back down.

ROLL DOWNS WITH DOUBLE FLOATING ARMS WITH WEIGHTS (LEVEL 4)

Use light weights up to 0.5kg (1.1lb). Remember, when you've rolled back up to standing, to take that moment to steady yourself before you raise your arms overhead.

WATCHPOINTS

→ Use appropriate core connection to control your alignment and movements.

ROLL DOWNS WITH DOUBLE FLOATING ARMS WITH WEIGHTS AND HEEL RAISE (LEVEL 5)

This brings everything together for greater challenge.

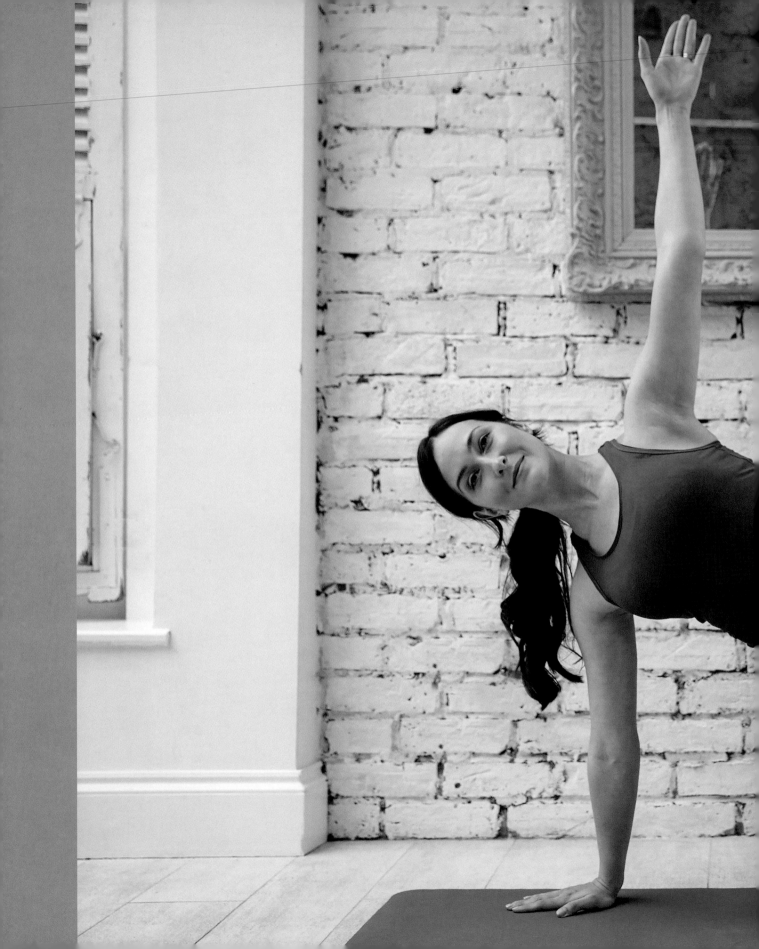

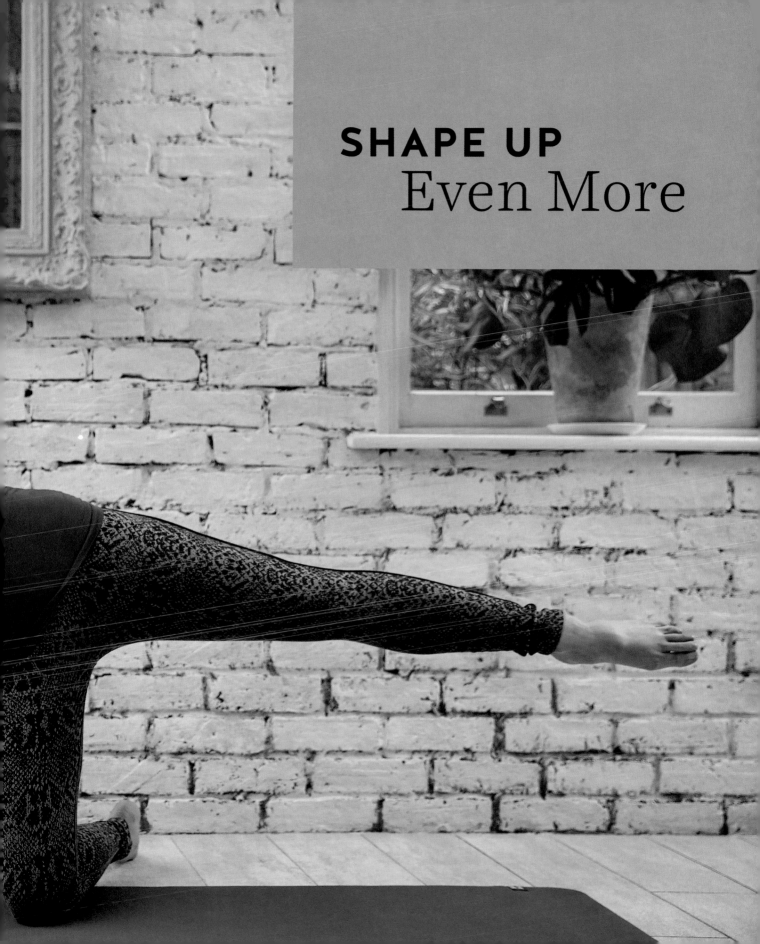

SHAPE UP
Even More

After mastering the New Fundamentals, work through this section of the book, which targets common problem areas: the abdominals, waist, buttocks, thighs and calves, arms and shoulders, and the back. Start to add the exercises into your workouts when you can do them confidently and with control. A balanced workout needs to include exercises from both the New Fundamentals and this section, and include the upper and lower body. You can include more exercises targeting a particular problem area, just don't overdo it. At the back of the book (see pages 197–218) you will find lots of balanced workouts of different lengths.

Abdominals

Classical Pilates features some of the best abdominal exercises ever created. You'll find them in this section with a few variations to challenge and motivate you. But, in truth, every exercise in this book is an abdominal exercise. If you work from your centre, you are sculpting your own natural in-built corset every time you practise.

OBLIQUE CURL UPS (LEVEL 2)

We introduced basic Curl Ups with variations on page 92. Here we look at a series of exercises to work your oblique abdominal muscles, which define your waistline.

STARTING POSITION
Relaxation Position (page 48), hands clasped behind the head with elbows open and within your peripheral vision.

ACTION
1 Breathe in to prepare.
2 Breathe out and nod your head, then continue to curl up sequentially through the neck centrally. Once your head is lifted in line with your shoulders, rotate your trunk to the right in a diagonal line. Direct your left rib to your right hip.
3 Breathe in and curl up further.
4 Breathe out and curl back down with control, reversing the diagonal line.
5 Repeat 5 times to each side. You can alternate or repeat to the same side if you prefer.

STARTING POSITION

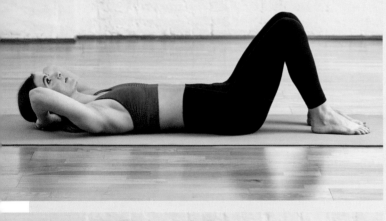

ACTION 2

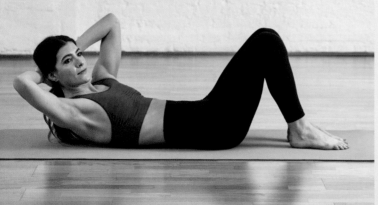

WATCHPOINTS

→ Use appropriate core connection to control your alignment and movements.

→ Try not to disturb your pelvis.

→ Keep your waist long on both sides.

→ Let your head remain heavy in the hands.

→ Keep your shoulders relaxed and down and away from your ears.

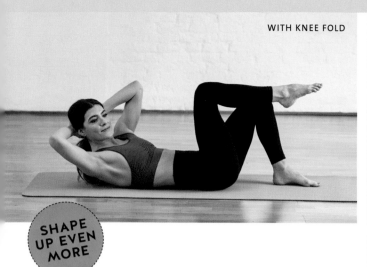

WITH KNEE FOLD

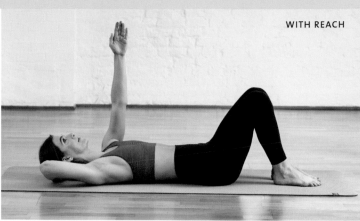

WITH REACH

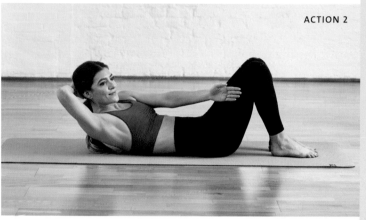

ACTION 2

OBLIQUE CURL UPS WITH KNEE FOLD (LEVEL 3)

We added lower-limb activity to Curl Ups (page 93), so now we will do the same with Oblique Curl Ups. As you curl to the right, fold your right knee in. Either repeat 5 times to one side then swap, or alternate sides.

OBLIQUE CURL UPS WITH REACH (LEVEL 3)

A slightly different Starting Position and an extra breath adds just that bit more challenge. Start with your right hand as in regular Oblique Curl Ups, your left hand raised above your shoulder, palm facing inward. As you curl up and across, reach your hand across, past the outside of your right knee. Take an extra breath and reach further, before coming back down. Keep your pelvis still and level. Either repeat 5 times to one side then swap sides, or alternate sides.

OBLIQUE CURL UPS WITH FURTHER REACH (LEVEL 4)

Follow the instructions above, but start with your left arm out slightly to the side, palm facing in. Start the Oblique Curl Up but bring the arm with you. Take an extra breath and reach further, before curling down to the Starting Position. Repeat up to 5 times, then swap arms and sides.

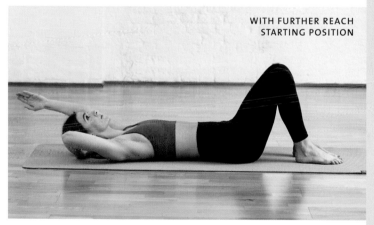

WITH FURTHER REACH STARTING POSITION

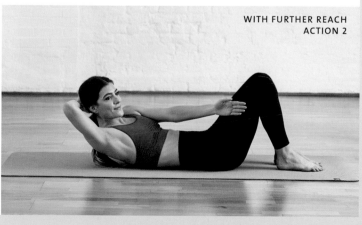

WITH FURTHER REACH ACTION 2

CRISS CROSS (LEVEL 5)

A challenging classical Pilates exercise, that's hard to get right (easy to get wrong!). It is worth putting in the hard work to build your strength and stamina because it gives a fabulous abdominal workout. Follow the directions closely to ensure you arrive in the curled-up Starting Position safely. Finish the exercise with equal precision.

STARTING POSITION

Relaxation Position (page 48). Lightly clasp both hands behind your head, keeping the elbows open, positioned just in front of your ears and within your peripheral vision. Double Knee Fold (page 70) one leg at a time with stability. Keeping your heels connected and your feet softly pointed, open your knees slightly. Breathe in wide and as you breathe out, nod your head and sequentially wheel your neck and upper body off the mat into a Curl Up Position (page 92).

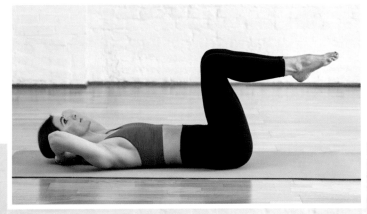

STARTING POSITION

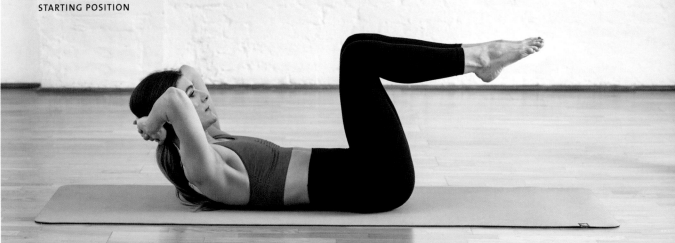

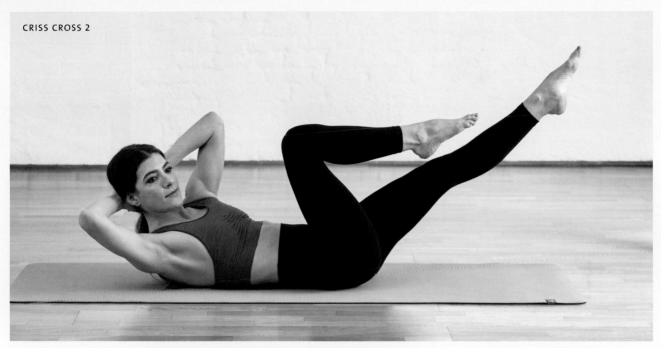

CRISS CROSS 2

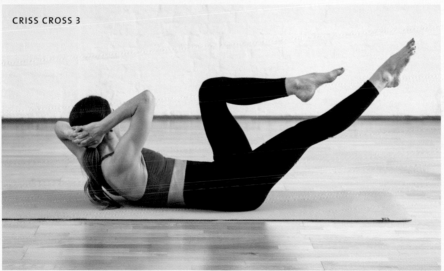

CRISS CROSS 3

ACTION

1 Breathe into the back of your ribcage as you hold the curled-up position.
2 Breathe out as you straighten and stretch your left leg away from you, simultaneously rotating your head and upper body to the right and drawing your right leg in further, toward your torso.

3 Breathe in as you draw your left leg back, simultaneously stretching your right leg away and rotating your upper body to the left.
4 Repeat up to 5 times.
5 Finally, draw both knees back in above your hips, and, with control, slowly curl back down and lower your feet, one at a time, with stability, to the mat.

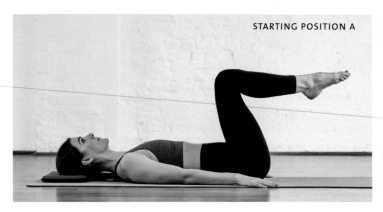

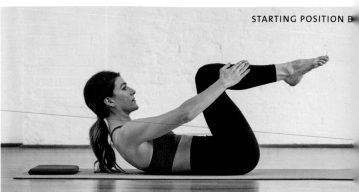

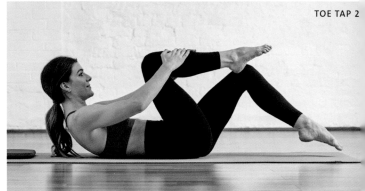

TOE TAP 2

SINGLE LEG STRETCH TOE TAPS (LEVEL 3)

The full classical Single Leg Stretch (opposite) requires both skill and stamina. This is useful preparation. Staying curled up will help you achieve the stamina, but if you feel any strain, come back down and practice regular Curl Ups to improve your abdominal strength.

STARTING POSITION

Relaxation Position (page 48). Double Knee Fold (page 70) one leg at a time with stability, allowing your thighs to rotate laterally (turn out) in the hip sockets. Softly point your feet. Breathe in wide and, as you breathe out, nod your head and sequentially wheel your neck and upper body off the mat into a Curl Up Position. Lengthen your arms forward and place your hands on the outside of your shins.

ACTION

1 Breathe into the back of your ribcage and curl up a little more.
2 Breathe out as you lower your left foot to the mat. Keep your knee bent and touch your toes to the mat first, simultaneously moving your left hand onto your right knee.
3 Breathe in and, maintaining your curled-up position, fold your leg up and in and return your left hand to your left shin.
4 Repeat on the other leg and hand.
5 Repeat up to 5 times before curling back down with control, returning the feet one at a time with stability.

WATCHPOINTS

→ Use appropriate core connection to control your alignment and movements.

→ Keep all your movements controlled, smooth and flowing.

→ Ensure that your pelvis remains undisturbed throughout; if necessary, stretch the leg away higher.

→ Focus on moving your legs independently from your pelvis and spine.

→ Don't lose the curl up!

→ Use your arms to draw your legs toward you, not to pull your spine up further.

→ Keep your focus on your abdominal area until you are ready to curl back down.

→ Maintain a slight turn-out of both legs throughout.

SINGLE LEG STRETCH (LEVEL 4)

The full classical version of this exercise remains one of the ultimate abdominal exercises – no argument.

STARTING POSITION

Relaxation Position (page 48). Double Knee Fold (page 70) one leg at a time with stability. Keeping your heels connected and your feet softly pointed, open your knees slightly. Breathe in wide to prepare. As you breathe out, nod your head and sequentially wheel your neck and upper body off the mat into a Curl Up Position (page 92). Lengthen your arms forward and place your hands on the outside of your shins.

ACTION

1 Breathe into the back of your ribcage as you hold the curled-up position.
2 Breathe out as you straighten your left leg forward, in line with the hip. Simultaneously move your left hand onto your right knee and gently draw your right leg in toward your torso.
3 Continue to breathe out as you switch legs, bending the left leg in and drawing it toward your torso as you press the right leg away. Your right hand is now on your left knee and your left hand on your left shin.
4 Breathe in as you repeat up to 5 times with each leg, pressing alternate legs away. Repeat up to 5 times before bringing both knees in toward your torso.
5 Roll your upper spine and head back to the mat. With stability, return your feet to the mat, one at a time.

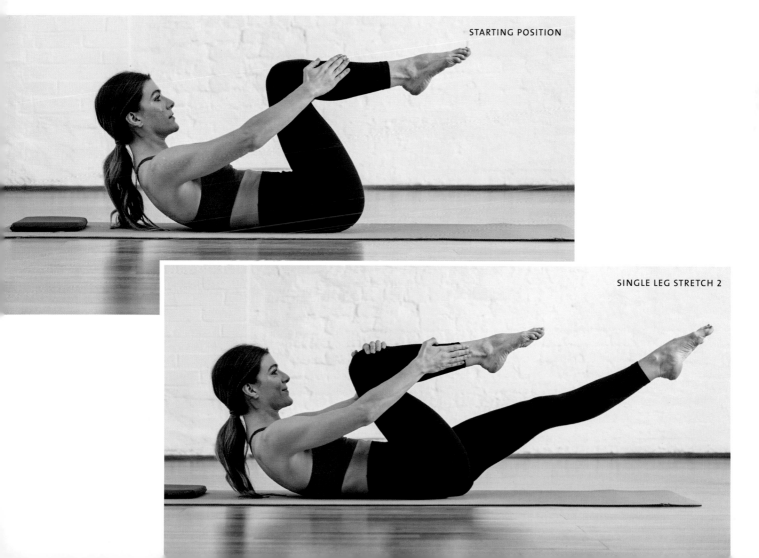

STARTING POSITION

SINGLE LEG STRETCH 2

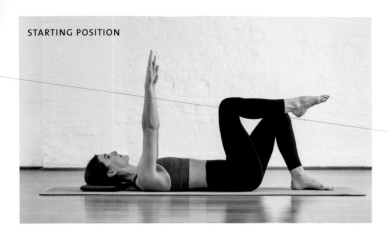

STARTING POSITION

DOUBLE LEG STRETCH PREP (LEVEL 2)

Practise this exercise to help develop the coordination and strength needed to perform the full classical Double Leg Stretch. It combines Ribcage Closure (page 79), Arm Circles (page 84) and Knee Folds (page 69) – and will really help to shape up your mid-section.

STARTING POSITION

Relaxation Position (page 48). Raise both arms above your shoulders, palms facing away. With stability, fold one knee in to a Single Knee Fold (page 69).

ACTION

1 Breathe in to prepare.
2 Breathe out as you simultaneously straighten your bent knee to 45 degrees and take both arms back into a Ribcage Closure (page 79).
3 Breathe in and circle your arms back around by your sides and up to the Starting Position as you bend your knee back in.
4 Repeat 4 times with this leg, then swap legs.

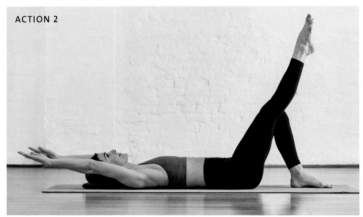

ACTION 2

ACTION 3

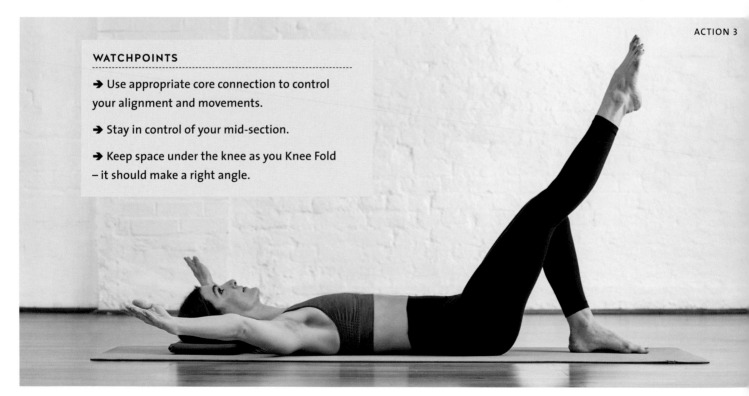

WATCHPOINTS

➜ Use appropriate core connection to control your alignment and movements.

➜ Stay in control of your mid-section.

➜ Keep space under the knee as you Knee Fold – it should make a right angle.

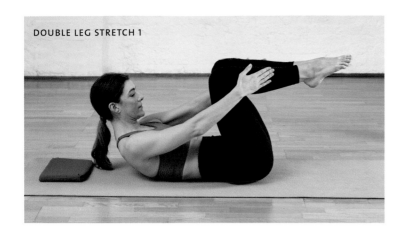

DOUBLE LEG STRETCH 1

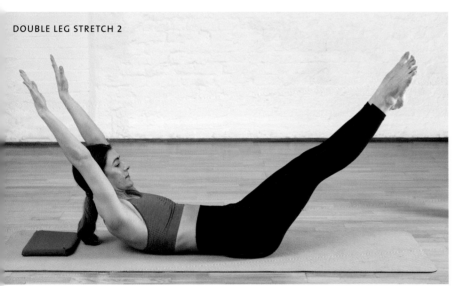

DOUBLE LEG STRETCH 2

WATCHPOINTS

➔ Keep all your movements controlled, smooth and flowing.

➔ Do not disturb the pelvis; let your legs move independently to your pelvis and spine.

➔ Move your arms and legs at the same time, creating opposition, length and openness across the front of your body.

➔ Keep the curl up.

➔ Focus down on your abdominal area.

➔ Do not over-reach with your arms.

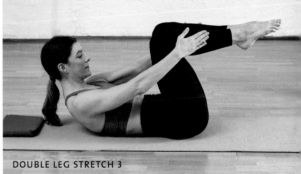

DOUBLE LEG STRETCH 3

DOUBLE LEG STRETCH (LEVEL 5)

Your abdominals will be amazing if you can master this classical exercise, which challenges by moving both the arms and legs away from your centre. A tough exercise, it develops strength and stamina alongside coordination and control. But we've prepared you well.

STARTING POSITION

Relaxation Position (page 48). Double Knee Fold (page 70) one leg at a time with stability. Keeping your heels connected and your feet softly pointed, open your knees slightly. Breathe in and as you breathe out, nod your head and wheel your neck and upper body off the mat into a Curl Up Position (page 92). Lengthen your arms forward and place your hands on the outside of your shins.

ACTION

1 Breathe in, remain curled up and straighten both legs, pressing them away from your body on a diagonal line. Connect your inner thighs and keep your legs turned out from the hips. Simultaneously reach your straight arms overhead, shoulder-width apart.

2 Breathe out as you bend the legs back in toward you, keeping the heels connected and knees open. Simultaneously circle your arms out to the side and around, to return back to the shins and draw the legs back to the Starting Position.

3 Repeat up to 10 times, then roll your upper spine and head back down to the mat. With stability, return your feet to the mat one at a time.

THE HUNDRED (LEVELS 1–5)

This energizing exercise sits at the heart of Joseph Pilates' original repertoire. Probably the most cardiovascular of his work, it is as much a breathing exercise as an abdominal exercise, boosting circulation and getting the heart pumping. We have given you five levels of difficulty. Work your way up gradually over time.

THE BREATHING PATTERN (LEVEL 1)

To connect mind and body, breathe in for 5 and out for 5. Work up to this by breathing in and out to a count of 3 and 4 initially.

WATCHPOINTS

➔ Use appropriate core connection to control your alignment and movements.

➔ Keep your shoulders and neck relaxed.

➔ Focus on your ribs closing down and drawing together during the exhalation and the progressive expansion of the ribcage during the inhalation.

STARTING POSITION
Relaxation Position (page 48). Place your hands on your lower ribcage.

ACTION

1 Breathe fully and deeply into the back and sides of your ribcage for up to a count of 5.

2 Breathe out completely up to a count of 5. Repeat 10 times. Stop if you feel dizzy.

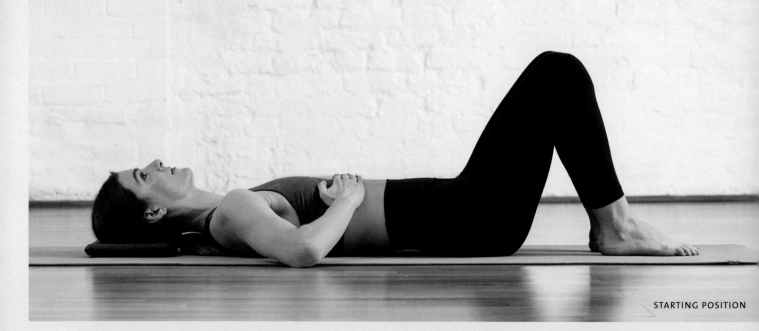

STARTING POSITION

THE HUNDRED: ADD A CURL UP AND ARM BEATS (LEVEL 2)

STARTING POSITION
Relaxation Position (page 48).

ACTION

1 Breathe in to prepare.
2 Breathe out, gently nod the head and Curl Up (page 92), raising both arms slightly off the mat.

3 Breathe in for a count of 5, staying curled up, as you beat your arms up and down 5 times. Focus on maintaining a connection of the core while breathing wide into the ribcage.
4 Breathe out for a count of 5, beating the arms 5 times.
5 Repeat up to 10 times, then still the arms, and slowly curl down with control.

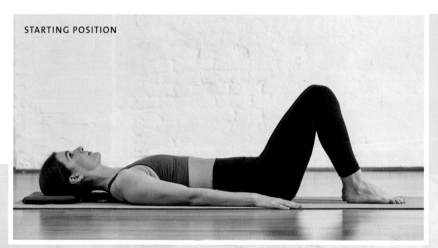

STARTING POSITION

WATCHPOINTS

→ Keep the pelvis stable and neutral.

→ Keep the waist long on both sides.

→ Initiate the pumping arm action from the shoulder joints, taking care not to flap your wrists.

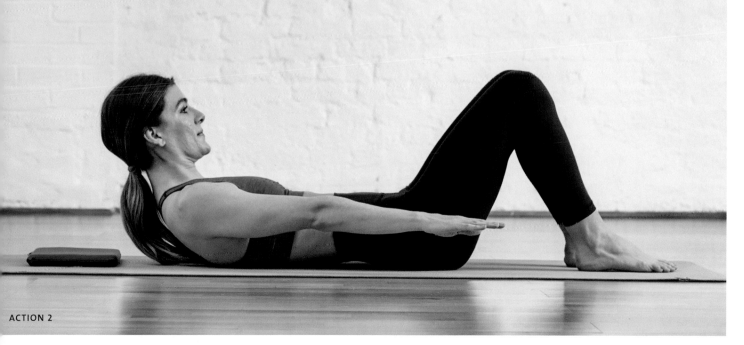

ACTION 2

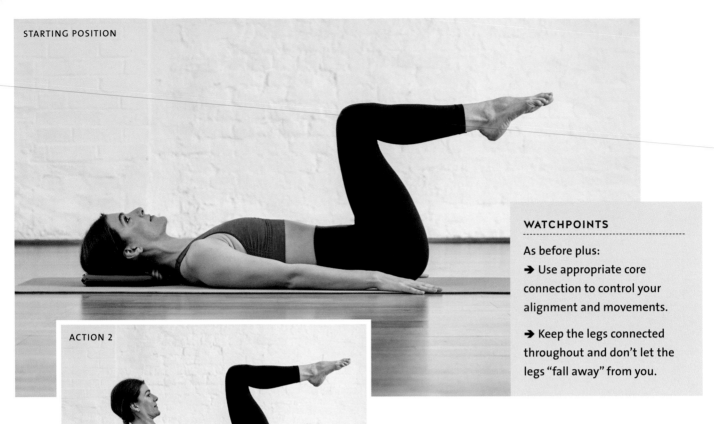

ACTION 2

THE HUNDRED WITH DOUBLE KNEE FOLD (LEVEL 3)

STARTING POSITION

Relaxation Position (page 48). Fold your knees up one at a time with stability into a Double Knee Fold position (page 70). Connect the inner thighs.

ACTION

1 Breathe in to prepare.
2 Breathe out as you nod your head and curl up, raising both arms off the mat.
3 Breathe in for a count of 5 as you beat your arms up and down 5 times.
4 Breathe out for a count of 5, beating the arms 5 times.
5 Repeat up to 10 times, then still the arms, curl back down with control and lower one foot at a time, with stability to the floor.

THE HUNDRED: STRAIGHT LEGS (LEVEL 4)

Straightening your legs adds an extra challenge for your core muscles. Keeping the legs together works your inner thighs, too.

STARTING POSITION

Relaxation Position (page 48). Fold your knees up a time with stability into a Double Knee Fold position (page 70). Connect the inner thighs.

ACTION

1 Breathe in to prepare.
2 Breathe out as you nod your head and curl up, raising both arms off the mat. Simultaneously straighten both legs to an angle of approximately 80 degrees to the mat. Your pelvis should remain undisturbed.
3 Breathe in for a count of 5 as you beat your arms up and down 5 times.
4 Breathe out for a count of 5, beating the arms 5 times.
5 Repeat up to 10 times, then still the arms, curl back down with control, bend your knees and lower one foot at a time, with stability, to the floor.

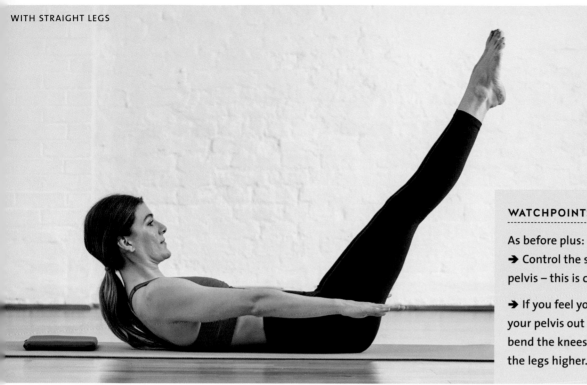

WATCHPOINTS

As before plus:
→ Control the stability of your pelvis – this is crucial.

→ If you feel your legs pulling your pelvis out of neutral, bend the knees and/or take the legs higher.

THE HUNDRED: STRAIGHT LEGS IN TURN-OUT (LEVEL 5)

Now the classical version of the exercise. The turned-out position of the legs means that you are also working your inner and outer thighs and deep buttock muscles. Follow all the instructions opposite, but when you bring your knees up into a Double Knee Fold Position (page 70), turn both legs out from the hips so the heels are connected and the knees hip-width apart. As you straighten your legs, maintain this turned out position.

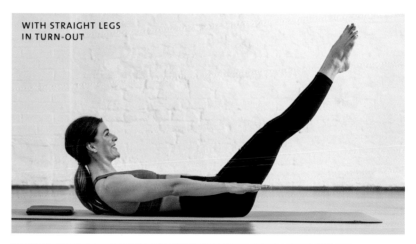

WITH STRAIGHT LEGS IN TURN-OUT

WATCHPOINTS

As before plus:
→ Try to focus on the inner thighs connecting.

→ Breathe into the back of the ribcage so that each inhalation helps you to maintain the curled-up position.

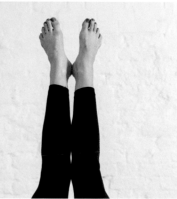

DIAMOND LEG LOWERS (LEVEL 4)

This exercise targets the abdominal and buttock muscles – and is harder than it looks.

STARTING POSITION

Relaxation Position (page 48). With stability, fold one knee up at a time into a Double Knee Fold Position (page 70). Cross your ankles and open your knees so your legs make a diamond shape.

Lightly clasp your hands behind each thigh (if you can't reach you can use a towel or scarf). Breathe in, then out as you nod your head and curl into a Curl Up (page 92). This is your starting position.

ACTION

1 Breathe in to prepare.
2 Breathe out and slowly lower both legs away from you. The diamond shape elongates. Keep holding your legs.
3 Breathe in and feel the thigh bones turning out and "wrapping around" in your buttocks.
4 Breathe out as you bring the legs back toward you.
5 Repeat up to 10 times, before curling back down and lowering one foot at a time to the floor with control.

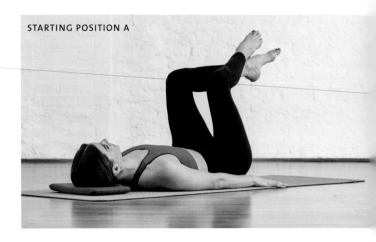

STARTING POSITION A

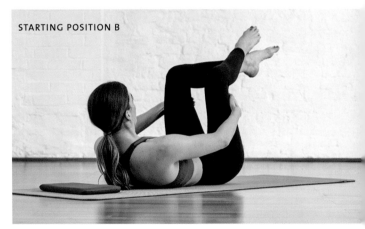

STARTING POSITION B

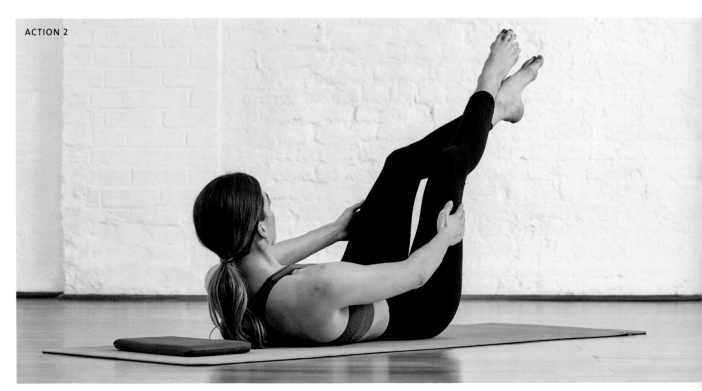

ACTION 2

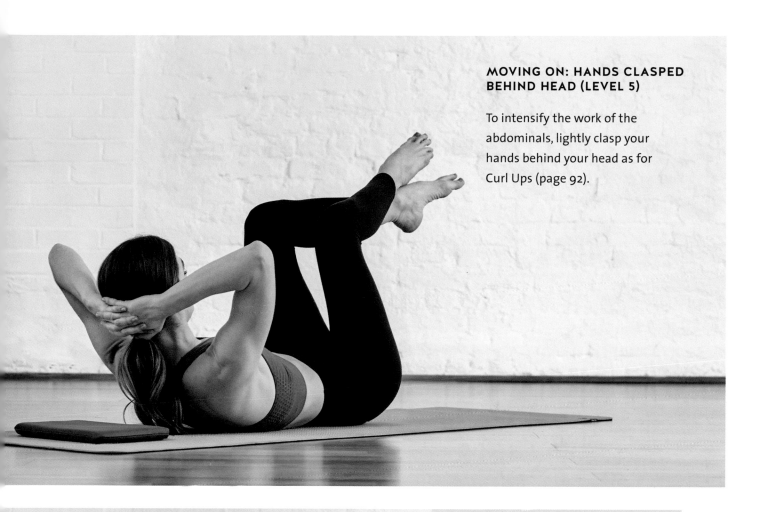

MOVING ON: HANDS CLASPED BEHIND HEAD (LEVEL 5)

To intensify the work of the abdominals, lightly clasp your hands behind your head as for Curl Ups (page 92).

ACTION 2

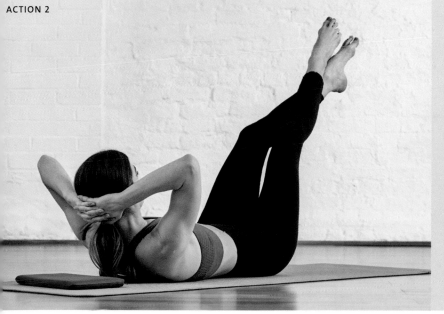

WATCHPOINTS

→ Use appropriate core connection to control your alignment and movements.

→ Keep your focus on your lower abdomen.

→ As you inhale, breathe into the back of the ribcage to help you stay curled up.

→ Stay in neutral pelvis when the legs move away and back.

→ Stop if you feel any discomfort in your neck. This means your abdominals aren't quite strong enough yet. Go back to Curl Ups and Oblique Curl Ups (page 116) before trying again.

THE PELVIC ROLL BACK SERIES

This series targets your abdominals and with some variations the arm muscles, too. If you can first master the C-Curve, Pelvic Roll Backs will seem much easier. We have given you some wonderful variations and combinations, nine in total!

PELVIC ROLL BACKS (LEVEL 3)

If you can master the C-Curve (page 94), it will make Pelvic Roll Backs seem much easier. We have given you nine brilliant variations and combinations in total.

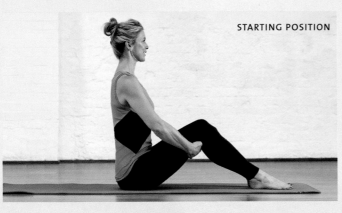

STARTING POSITION

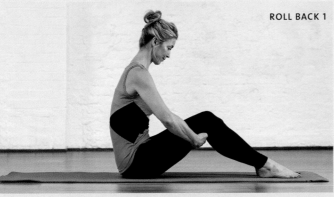

ROLL BACK 1

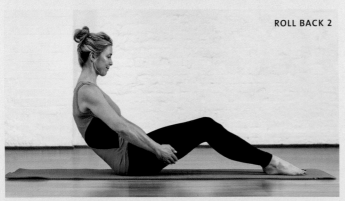

ROLL BACK 2

WATCHPOINTS

➜ Use appropriate core connection to control your alignment and movements.

➜ Once the C-Curve has been established, it is the pelvis rolling away from the legs that creates the movement.

➜ Roll directly through your centre-line.

STARTING POSITION

Sit tall at the front of your mat, legs bent and hip-width apart, feet grounded on the mat. Initially you can place your hands around the backs of your thighs for support, but work toward holding the arms in front of you, just below shoulder-height.

ACTION

1 Breathe in as you lengthen the spine in a C-Curve (page 94), shoulders over hips.
2 Breathe out as you roll the pelvis, tailbone curling toward the pubic bone, until the back of your pelvis is supported by the mat.
3 Breathe in as you maintain your roll-back position, ensuring the spine is still in a C-Curve; your elbows will bend.
4 Breathe out as you initiate with your head and roll the C-Curved spine forward, returning your shoulders over your hips. Then, moving your pelvis and head simultaneously, lengthen your spine back to upright.
5 Repeat up to 5 times.

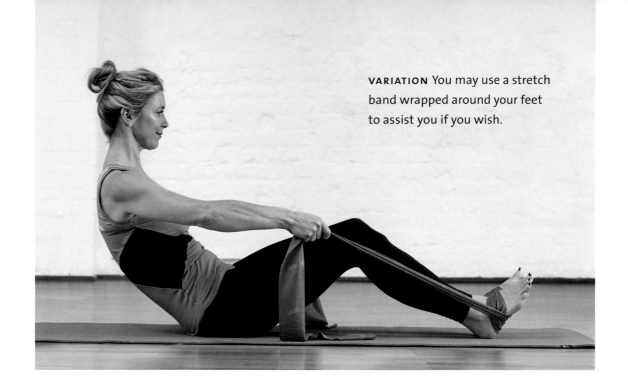

VARIATION You may use a stretch band wrapped around your feet to assist you if you wish.

PELVIC ROLL BACKS WITH LEG SLIDE (LEVEL 3)

Adding a leg action increases the challenge.

STARTING POSITION
As for Pelvic Roll Backs (opposite), hands held out in front.

ACTION
Follow Action Points 1–3 for Pelvic Roll Backs, then:

4 Breathe out and slide one foot in toward your hip (it won't slide far).
5 Breathing in, slide the foot back to the Starting Position.
6 Repeat up to 3 times with each foot before rolling back up.

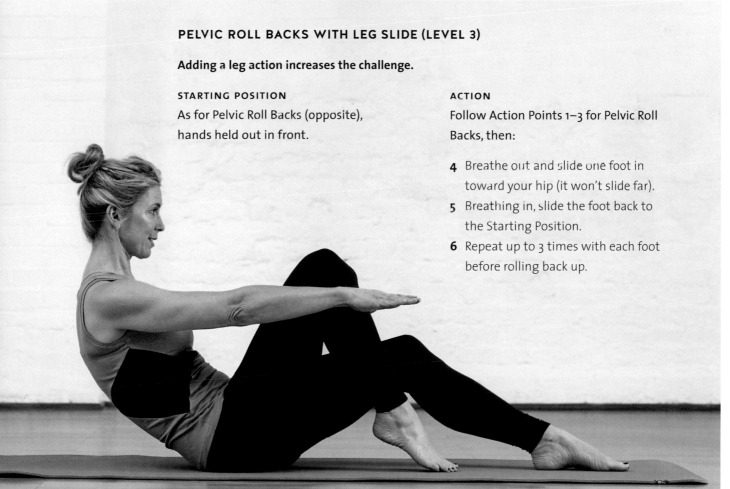

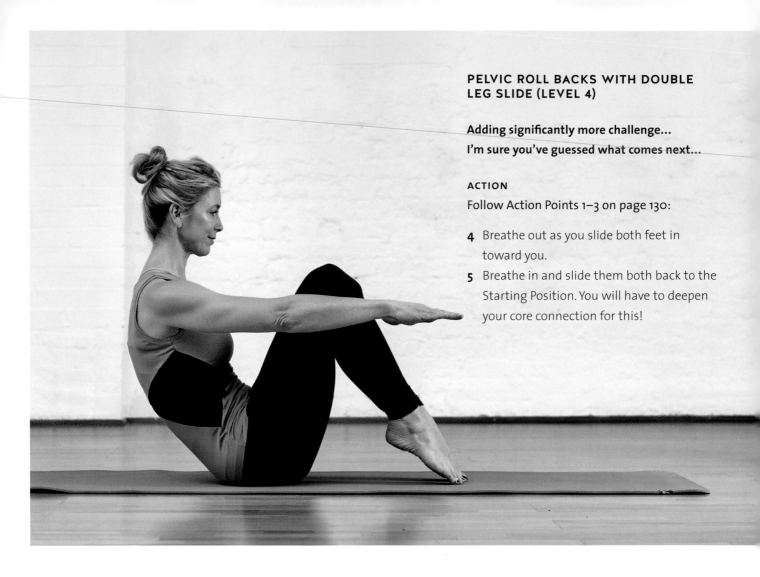

PELVIC ROLL BACKS WITH DOUBLE LEG SLIDE (LEVEL 4)

Adding significantly more challenge...
I'm sure you've guessed what comes next...

ACTION
Follow Action Points 1–3 on page 130:

4 Breathe out as you slide both feet in toward you.
5 Breathe in and slide them both back to the Starting Position. You will have to deepen your core connection for this!

PELVIC ROLL BACKS WITH KNEE FOLD (LEVEL 4)

These are difficult exercises, so take a break between repetitions if necessary. The Watchpoints apply to all the Roll Back variations.

STARTING POSITION
As for Pelvic Roll Backs (page 130), hands held out in front.

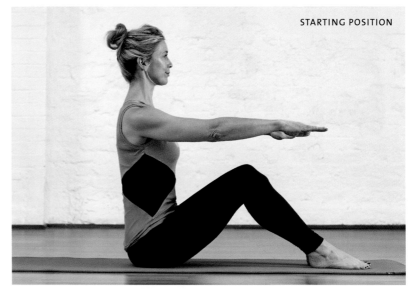

STARTING POSITION

ACTIONS 2–3

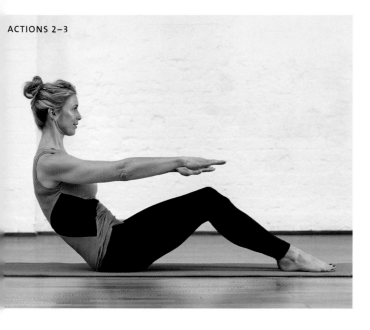

ACTION

Follow Action Points 1–3 for Pelvic Roll Backs, then:

4 Breathe out and fold one knee in toward you.

5 Breathing in, replace the foot.

6 Repeat 3 times with each knee, then roll back up as on page 130.

ADD A KNEE FOLD

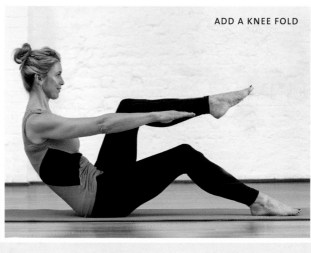

KNEE FOLD AND EXTEND (LEVEL 5)

Harder still, knee fold and extend the leg to add even more challenge.

WATCHPOINTS

➔ Use appropriate core connection to control your alignment and movements.

➔ Ensure your C-Curve remains lengthened through all the exercises.

➔ Try to keep your feet, or foot grounded throughout.

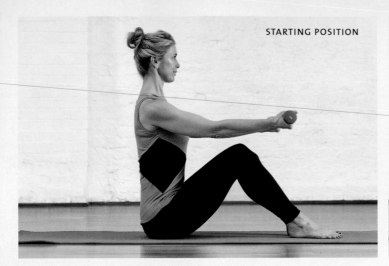

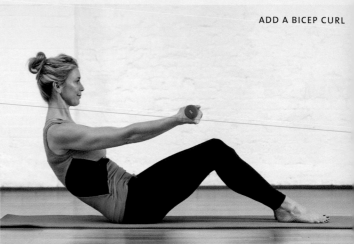

PELVIC ROLL BACKS WITH BICEP CURLS (LEVEL 4)

Here we have added weights to create some arm work. You will need a long, light stretch band or two light hand weights, initially no more than 0.5kg (1.1lb) each.

STARTING POSITION

Sit tall on your mat as for Pelvic Roll Backs (page 130). Either take one weight in each hand or wrap the stretch band around each foot and hold one end firmly in each hand. Have your palms facing upward, shoulders open.

ACTION

Follow Action Points 1–3 for Pelvic Roll Backs, then:

4 Breathe out and bend both elbows in a Bicep Curl; maintain the roll back.

5 Breathe out and straighten your arms.

6 Breathe in and roll back up.

7 Repeat up to 6 times. If you prefer, do more Bicep Curls in the rolled-back position before rolling up.

SIMULTANEOUS SINGLE LEG SLIDE (LEVEL 4)

Harder still, roll and slide.

WATCHPOINTS

→ Use appropriate core connection to control your alignment and movements.

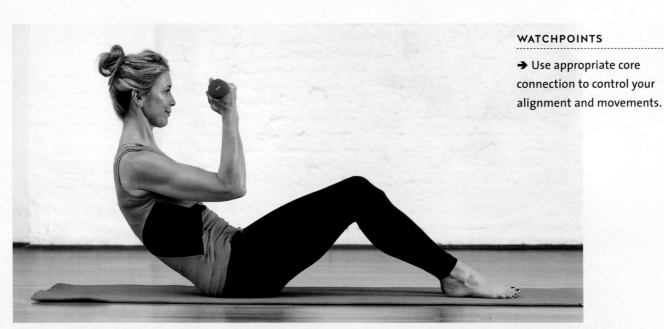

PELVIC ROLL BACKS WITH ROWING PREP (LEVEL 4)

This targets the biceps again and, of course, the abdominals. It's adapted from the arm work on a Pilates Reformer machine in the studio. You will need a long, light stretch band or two light hand weights, initially no more than 0.5kg (1.1lb).

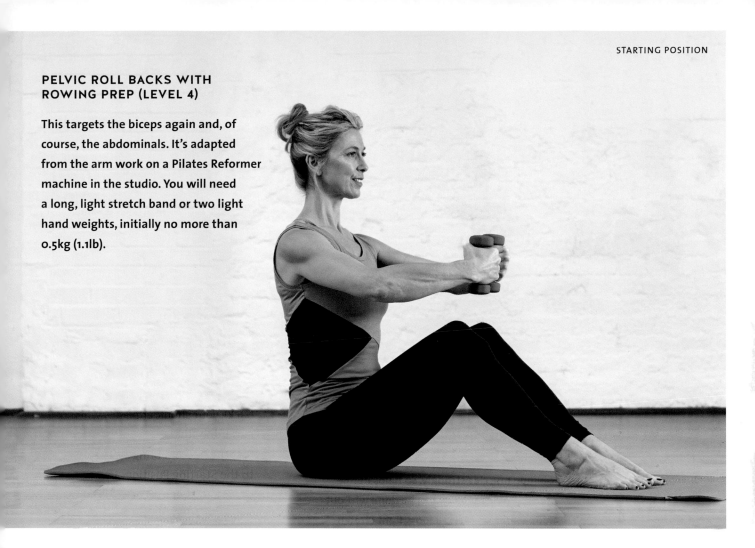

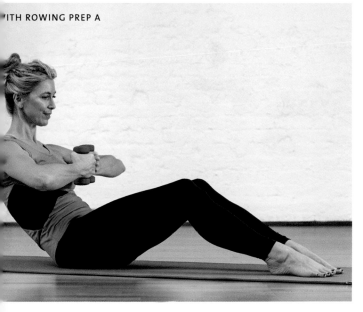

WITH ROWING PREP A

STARTING POSITION

As for Pelvic Roll Backs (page 130), holding your weights or band, arms out just below shoulder-height, circled in front of you, elbows bent, palms facing toward you.

ACTION

Follow Action Points 1–3 for Pelvic Roll Backs, then:

4 Breathe out and bend your elbows, bringing your palms in toward you.
5 Breathe in and hold the position.
6 Breathe out and roll back up returning your arms to the Starting Position.
7 Repeat up to 6 times. You could do more arm curls in the roll-back position, before rolling back up.

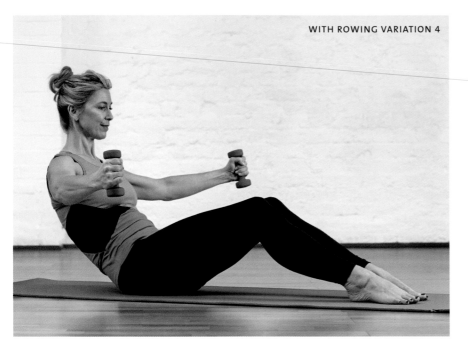

PELVIC ROLL BACKS WITH ROWING VARIATION (LEVEL 4)

Your upper arms and the backs of your shoulders do the work in this variation – and the abdominals again, of course. You will need a long, light stretch band or two light hand weights, initially no more than 0.5kg (1.1lb).

STARTING POSITION
As for Pelvic Roll Backs (page 130).

ACTION
Follow Action Points 1–3 for Pelvic Roll Backs, then:

4   Breathe in and open your arms to the side (if using a band, gently pull back); your shoulder blades will move closer together.
5   Breathe out and bring your arms back to the Starting Position.
6   Breathe in and roll back up.
7   Repeat up to 6 times.

PELVIC ROLL BACKS, ROWING PREP WITH ROTATION (LEVEL 5)

This version works your oblique muscles strongly, so helps define your waist. It is easier with a stretch band but can be done without if you have strong abdominals. You will need a long, light stretch band or two light hand weights, initially no more than 0.5kg (1.1lb).

STARTING POSITION
As for Pelvic Roll Backs (page 130). Have your arms out in front of you, just below shoulder-height, palms facing inward, elbows bent and shoulders open.

ACTION
Follow Action Points 1–3 for Pelvic Roll Backs, then:

4   Breathe out and open your right arm, simultaneously rotating your trunk to the right.
5   Breathe in and rotate back to face forward; your arm moves back with you.
6   Repeat up to 5 times to each side, then breathe out to roll back up.

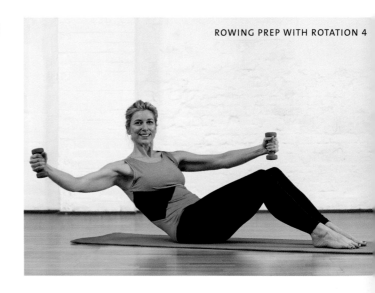

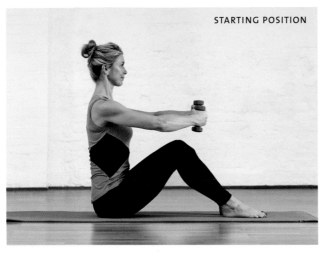

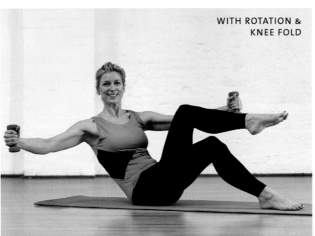

WITH ROTATION &
KNEE FOLD

PELVIC ROLL BACKS, ROTATE AND KNEE FOLD (LEVEL 6)

Yes, we have spent hours locked away in a room coming up with ways to challenge you!

STARTING POSITION

As for Pelvic Roll Backs (page 130).

ACTION

Follow Action Points 1–3 for Pelvic Roll Backs, then:

4 When you rotate to the right, lift your left foot from the mat.

5 Return the foot to the mat before you centre, then rotate to the left, lifting your right foot.

6 Return the foot to the mat and return to centre before rolling back up.

7 Repeat up to 5 times, then breathe out to roll back up.

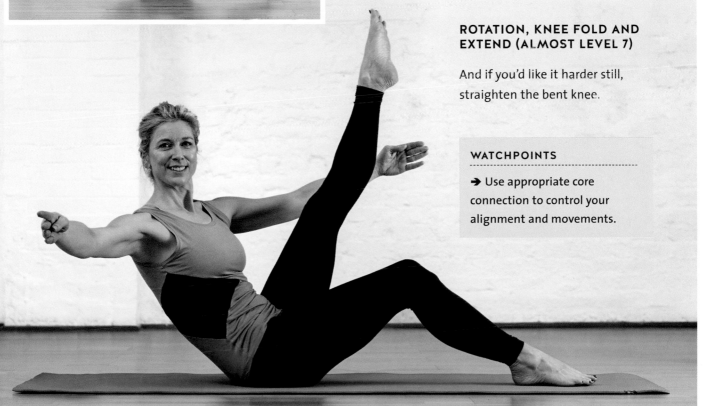

ROTATION, KNEE FOLD AND EXTEND (ALMOST LEVEL 7)

And if you'd like it harder still, straighten the bent knee.

WATCHPOINTS

→ Use appropriate core connection to control your alignment and movements.

Waist

All the abdominal exercises also target the waist, but in this section, we are looking to define and streamline it even further. To work the waist muscles, we need to work the oblique muscles and also muscles that bend your spine to the side, which we do with these Rolls, Reaches, Twists and Lifts.

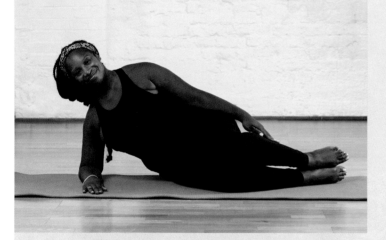

STARTING POSITION

SIDE TWIST SERIES

SIDE TWIST PREP (LEVEL 3)

This is the first in this series of exercises targeting both the waist and the shoulders.

STARTING POSITION

Lie on your right side with your right arm bent, elbow directly beneath your shoulder and forearm directed forward. Bend your knees with the thighs either back in line with your hips or bent so your feet line up with your spine (as for Oyster, page 87) whichever suits you best. Connect your inner thighs and lengthen your top arm along the top of your left leg.

ACTION

1 Breathe in to prepare, and lift the pelvis off the mat so the trunk makes one long diagonal line. Simultaneously float your left arm up and over your head.

2 Breathe out as you lower your pelvis and hips down with control to return to the Starting Position.

3 Repeat 5 times on both sides.

WATCHPOINTS

➜ Use appropriate core connection to control your alignment and movements.

➜ Stay in one long line.

➜ Keep the legs actively connected throughout.

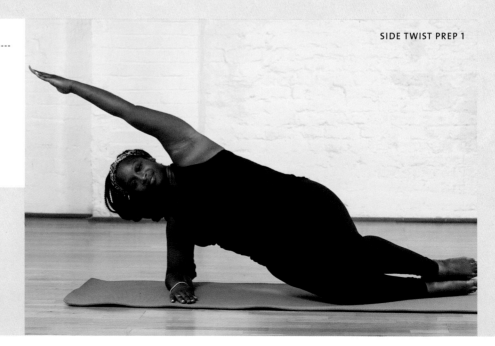

SIDE TWIST PREP 1

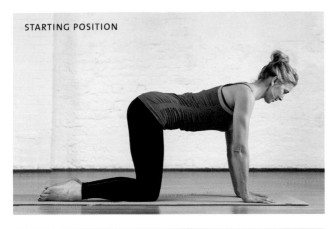

DYNAMIC SIDE TWIST PREP 2

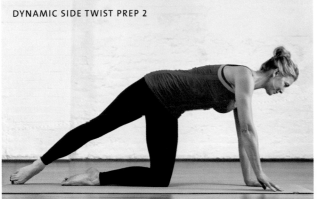

DYNAMIC SIDE TWIST PREP (LEVEL 4)

A fun exercise to tone your waist, upper arms, shoulders, buttocks and hips. It challenges your core stability and also works on your balance (you may wobble at first). There's quite a lot to take in when you first try this exercise so study the photos carefully and read the instructions several times.

STARTING POSITION
Four-point Kneeling (page 54). Take a moment to ensure your hands are beneath your shoulders, knees beneath your hips and spine lengthened.

WATCHPOINTS

➜ Use appropriate core connection to control your alignment and movements.

➜ Keep both sides of your waist lengthened at all times.

➜ Keep your head in line with your spine.

➜ At each stage take a moment to check your alignment.

ACTION

1 Breathe in wide to prepare and transfer your weight onto your left hand and knee.
2 As you breathe out, rotate your trunk to the right, simultaneously straighten your right leg away, foot sliding along the floor in line with your body. You may need to swivel on your knee to do this. Your right arm lifts up in line with your shoulders.
3 Breathe in and stay lengthened facing forwards.
4 Breathe out as you return, with control, to the Starting Position.
5 Repeat 5 times alternating sides.

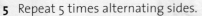

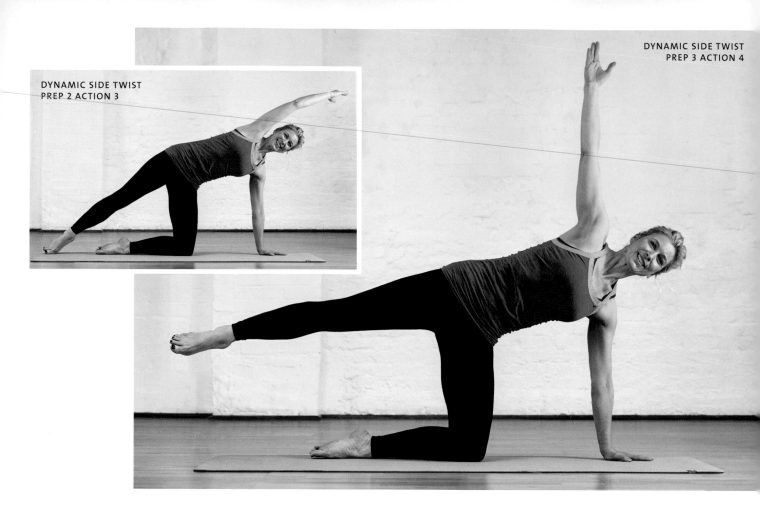

DYNAMIC SIDE TWIST
PREP 2 ACTION 3

DYNAMIC SIDE TWIST
PREP 3 ACTION 4

DYNAMIC SIDE TWIST PREP 2 (LEVEL 5)

STARTING POSITION

As Dynamic Side Twist Prep.

ACTION

Follow Action Point 1 for Dynamic Side
Twist Prep, but this time:

2 As your trunk rotates, take your top arm up
   and overhead, reaching in line with your body,
   lengthening from fingers to toes.
3 Breathe in, maintaining the length in your trunk.
4 Breathe out as you return to the Starting Position
   with control.
5 Repeat 5 times to each side alternating sides.

DYNAMIC SIDE TWIST PREP 3 (LEVEL 5)

This is getting seriously challenging.

STARTING POSITION

As Dynamic Side Twist Prep.

ACTION

Follow Action Points 1–3 for Dynamic Side Twist Prep,
then:

4 Breathe out and lift the top leg to hip-height, in line
   with your trunk. You are now balanced on your hand,
   knee and lower leg. Stay strong in your centre.
5 Breathe in and lower the leg as you circle your
   arm back.
6 Breathe out as you return to the Starting Position
   with control.
7 Repeat 5 times to each side.

SIDE KICK SERIES

SMALL CIRCLES (LEVEL 3)

In a side-lying exercise you may think it's all about the legs, but in fact your waist has to work hard to keep you stable. If you put your hand on your waist for a moment while practising, you'll feel the muscles working away. No wonder we say Pilates is top-to-toe conditioning.

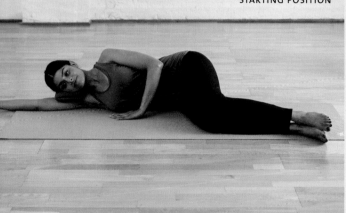

STARTING POSITION

STARTING POSITION

Lie on your right side in a Chair Position (page 57), stacking shoulders, hips and ankles. Place your left hand on the mat in front of you and bend the elbow to lightly support you.

ACTION

1 Breathe in to prepare.
2 Breathe out and lift and straighten your top leg, bringing it back, in parallel, so that it is hip-height in line with your spine. Softly point your foot.
3 Breathe in as you begin to circle the leg around, forward, up, back and down to the Starting Position.
4 Breathe out, then repeat another circle in the same direction.
5 Repeat up to 5 times in the same direction (1 breath for each circle) and then reverse direction.

Repeat up to 10 times and then turn over to repeat on the other side.

WATCHPOINTS

➔ Use appropriate core connection to control your alignment and movements.

➔ The circle is small, about the size of a watermelon. The centre of your circle should be in a line with your hip joint.

➔ Keep your waist lifted and lengthened evenly on both sides.

➔ Keep your chest open and your focus directly ahead of you.

➔ Make sure that your pelvis remains stable throughout.

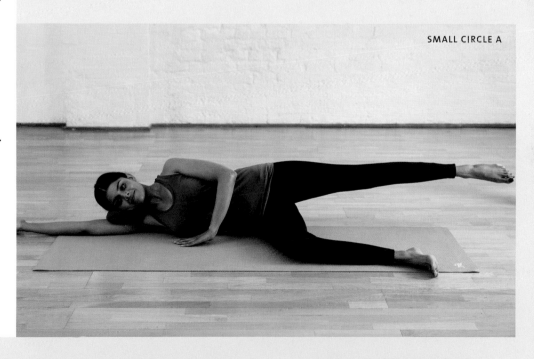

SMALL CIRCLE A

TORPEDO PREP (LEVEL 3)

One of my personal favourites, this exercise really hits the spot. You'll feel your waist working to keep you stable.

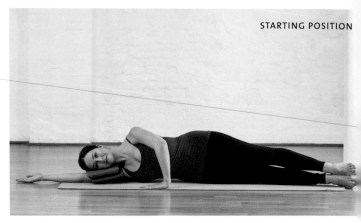

STARTING POSITION

Lie on your right side in a straight line, stacking your shoulders, hips and ankles. Lengthen your legs away from you, either in line with your spine or forward at a slight angle, keeping your legs in parallel and softly point your feet. Lengthen your right arm beneath your head and in line with your spine. Place your left hand on the mat in front of your ribcage and bend your elbow to lightly support your position.

ACTION 2 – ADD A LEG LIFT

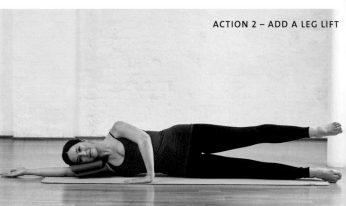

WATCHPOINTS

→ Use appropriate core connection to control your alignment and movements.

→ Lengthen as you lift your legs.

→ Keep your waist equally long on both sides.

→ Focus on preventing your spine from rolling forward or back.

→ Keep your legs in parallel, knees facing forward.

→ Lift and lower the legs on one plane only; do not allow them to drift forward or back.

→ Keep your chest open, and your focus directly ahead of you.

ACTION

1 Breathe in to prepare.
2 Breathe out and lift your top leg as high as you can without disturbing your pelvis.
3 Breathe in and lift the lower leg to meet the top leg.
4 Breathe out and squeeze both legs together as you lower both back down.

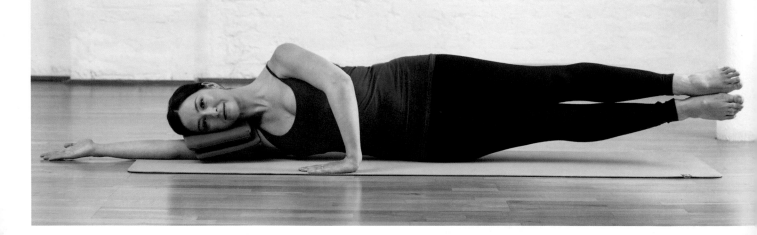

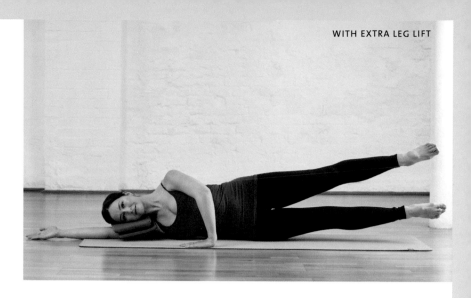

SHAPE UP EVEN MORE

TORPEDO (LEVEL 3)

Though you may find it a little harder to lift both legs together, we've kept this as a Level 3 exercise because the challenge to your stability is very similar to the Torpedo Prep.

Follow the directions for Torpedo Prep (opposite), but breathe out and lift both legs at the same time, keeping your inner thighs connected. Breathe in and lower both legs with control.

TORPEDO WITH HAMSTRING CURL (LEVEL 4)

Follow the directions for Torpedo above, then:

3 Still breathing out, bend both knees in a speedy, but controlled, hamstring curl.
4 Breathe in, straighten both legs again, and lower both legs with control.

TORPEDO WITH EXTRA LEG LIFT (LEVEL 4)

Follow the directions for Torpedo, then:

3 Breathe in, hold the position of the underneath leg and slightly raise your top leg even further.
4 Breathe out and raise your underneath leg to join your top leg; connect the inner thighs.
5 Breathe in and, still squeezing, lower your legs with control back to the mat.
6 Repeat up to 10 times, then change sides.

TORPEDO (LEVEL 5)

For an additional challenge, lengthen your arms above your head.

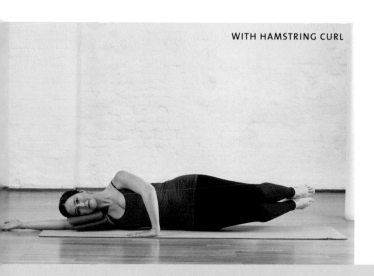

WITH HAMSTRING CURL

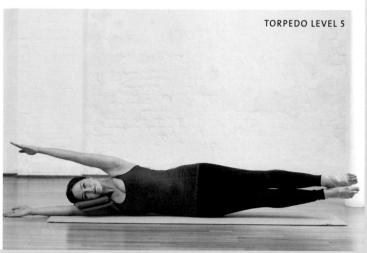

TORPEDO LEVEL 5

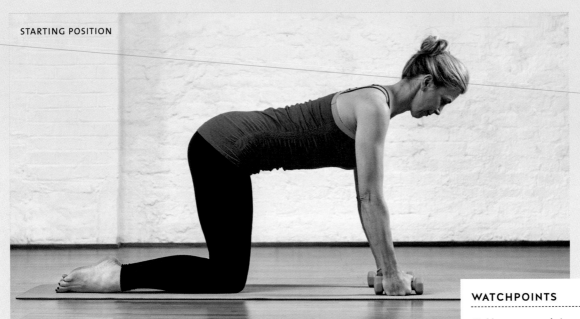

Arms & shoulders

We have included a wide variety of ways to reach the upper arms in this section of the book, including using your bodyweight, stretch bands and hand-held weights.

FOUR-POINT KNEELING FLIES (LEVEL 3)

Here we are working towards combining Table Top (page 74) with Flies (opposite). As with all the one-sided work, the challenge is to stay central and not twist. This means your obliques have to work extra hard, exercising the waist as well as well as the arms and upper body (and buttocks when you lift the leg). You will need two light hand weights, no more than 0.5kg (1.1lb).

STARTING POSITION

Four-point Kneeling (page 54), but hold the weights in each hand, palms facing inward. You will be on your knuckles. (If this is not comfortable place the weights close by your hands to pick up as needed.)

FOUR POINT KNEELING FLIES A

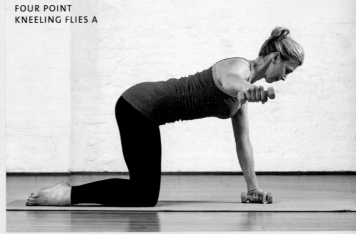

ACTION

1 Breathe in, preparing your body to move.
2 Breathe out and open one arm to the side in a Fly action. Keep the arm lengthened but retain its natural curve.
3 Breathe in and return to the Starting Position.
4 Repeat up to 8 times with each arm.

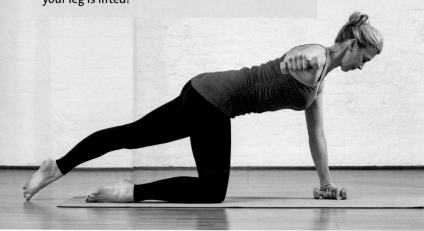

SHAPE UP EVEN MORE

TABLE TOP WITH FLIES (LEVEL 4)

To make this more challenging, we can reduce your base of support. Slide one leg away along the mat in line with your hip (as for Table Top, page 74), and then lift the opposite arm in a Fly action. Keep your softly pointed foot in contact with the mat. Do not disturb the pelvis or spine. Keep your foot on the mat.

Repeat 4 Flies with the same arm before sliding the foot back to the Starting Position. Then swap arms and legs.

TABLE TOP WITH WEIGHTS AND LIFTED LEG (LEVEL 5)

When you feel ready, challenge your balance and core stability even more by doing the Flies with a lifted leg.

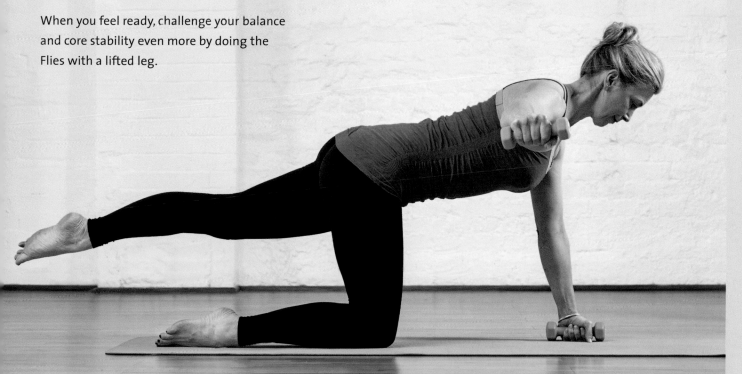

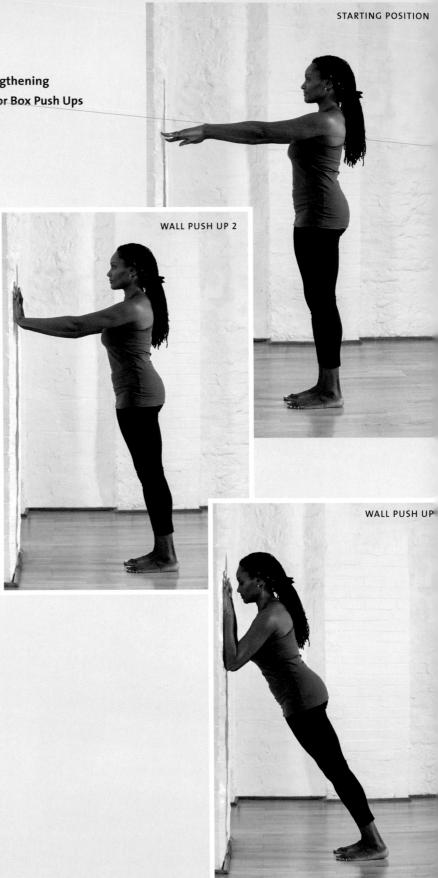

WALL PUSH UPS (LEVEL 2)

A gentle but highly effective exercise for strengthening the arms, this is also the perfect preparation for Box Push Ups (page 150).

STARTING POSITION
Stand tall, facing a wall, far enough away that only your fingertips touch. Have your arms just lower than shoulder-width apart and feet hip-width apart.

ACTION
1 Breathe in to prepare.
2 Breathe out as you bend your elbows down, rolling sequentially through your wrists and hands to lean your body toward the wall. Move your trunk as one piece, keeping your body straight.
3 Breathe in to hold the position.
4 Breathe out as you press back out to the starting position.
5 Repeat 8 times.

WALL PUSH UP 2

WATCHPOINTS

➜ Use appropriate core connection to control your alignment and movements.

➜ Keep your body long and strong; do not collapse in the middle, keep your ribs connected.

➜ Bend your elbows downward but stay open across your collarbones.

➜ Keep your head and neck in line with the rest of your body.

➜ Hinge from your ankle joint to achieve the right movement.

WALL PUSH UP

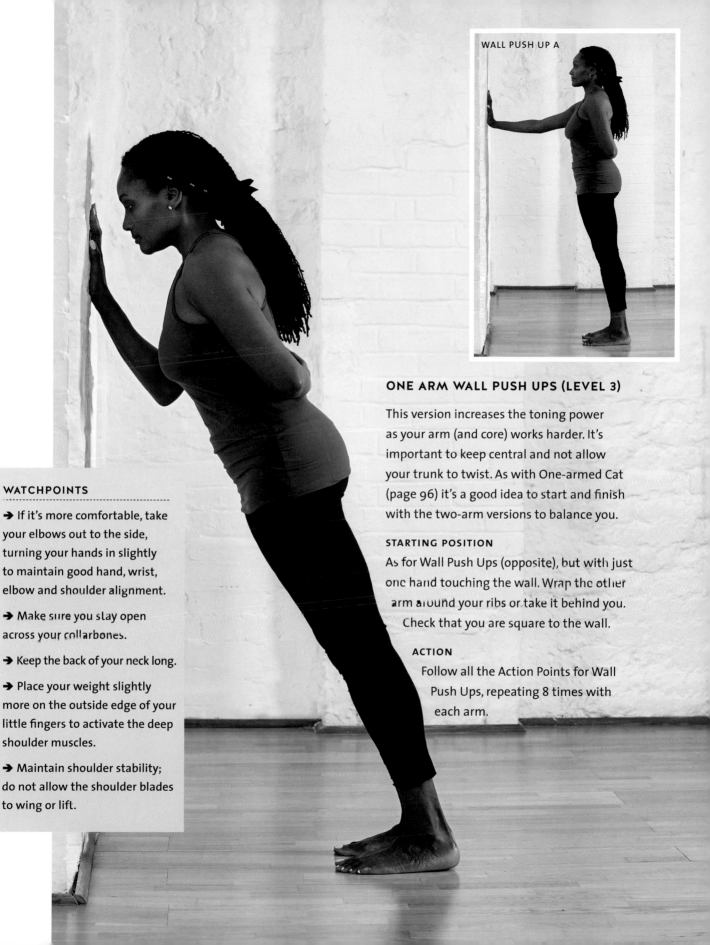

ONE ARM WALL PUSH UPS (LEVEL 3)

This version increases the toning power as your arm (and core) works harder. It's important to keep central and not allow your trunk to twist. As with One-armed Cat (page 96) it's a good idea to start and finish with the two-arm versions to balance you.

STARTING POSITION

As for Wall Push Ups (opposite), but with just one hand touching the wall. Wrap the other arm around your ribs or take it behind you. Check that you are square to the wall.

ACTION

Follow all the Action Points for Wall Push Ups, repeating 8 times with each arm.

WATCHPOINTS

➔ If it's more comfortable, take your elbows out to the side, turning your hands in slightly to maintain good hand, wrist, elbow and shoulder alignment.

➔ Make sure you stay open across your collarbones.

➔ Keep the back of your neck long.

➔ Place your weight slightly more on the outside edge of your little fingers to activate the deep shoulder muscles.

➔ Maintain shoulder stability; do not allow the shoulder blades to wing or lift.

LEG PULL FRONT PREP (LEVEL 4)

Top-to-toe conditioning Pilates style. Do not think of this as a "holding" exercise – it is not a plank. You build strength by controlling your alignment and movement. You'll probably need to turn your Dimmer Switch up (page 64) to stop your pelvis and spine dipping toward the mat.

STARTING POSITION
Four-point Kneeling (page 54).

ACTION

1 Breathe in to prepare.
2 Breathe out and slide your right leg along the mat in line with your hip joint. Tuck your toes under and take the weight on the ball of the foot. Keep your trunk stable, but you may need to transfer your weight a little to stay centred.
3 Breathing in, slide your left leg away.
4 Breathe out and check your weight is evenly balanced between your hands and feet.
5 Breathe in and press back through your heels; your trunk will simultaneously shift backward. Maintain one long line from head to heels.

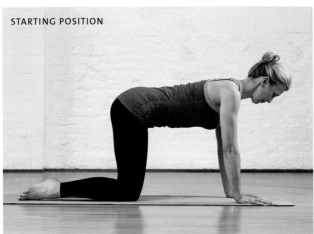

STARTING POSITION

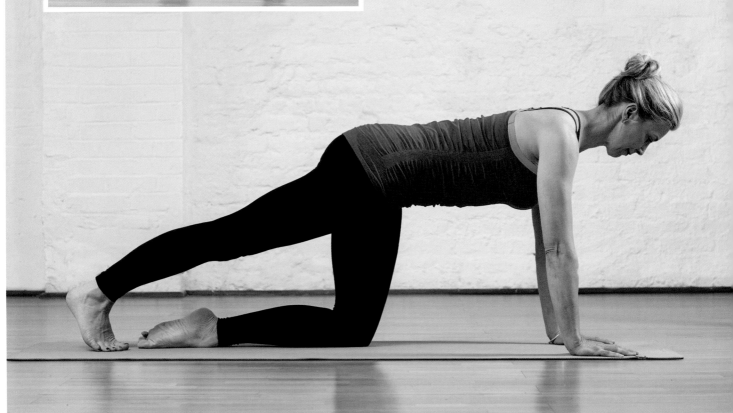

ACTION 2

6 Breathe out as you bring your weight forward again, shoulders directly over wrists.

7 Repeat 3 times, then breathe in as you bend your left knee, sliding the foot back to the Starting Position.

8 Breathe out and repeat with the right leg.

9 Work up to 4 repetitions of the sequence, alternating your starting leg.

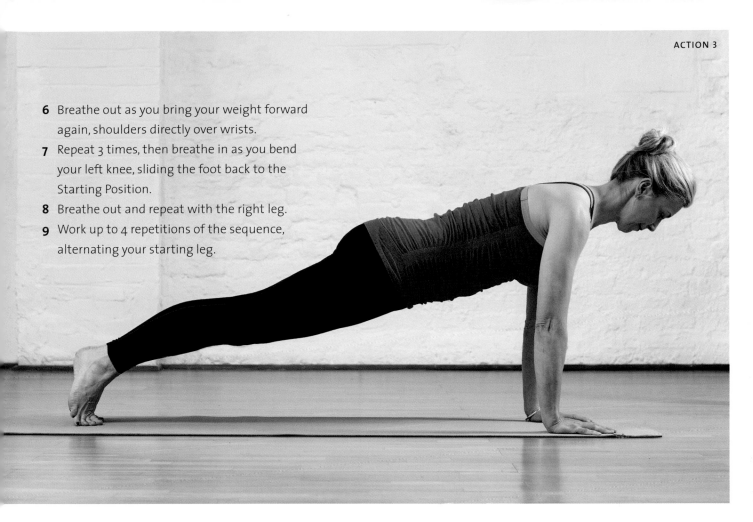

WATCHPOINTS

→ Use appropriate core connection to control your alignment and movements.

→ As you press your heel to the mat, continue to lengthen out through the crown of your head.

→ Keep your shoulder blades connected to the back of your ribcage. Lift the weight of your body away from your arms and keep your chest open.

→ Keep both arms and legs fully lengthened throughout, without locking your elbows or knees.

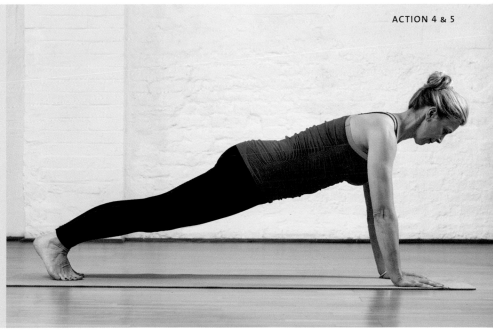

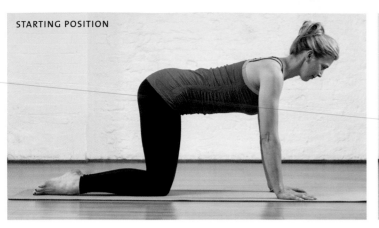

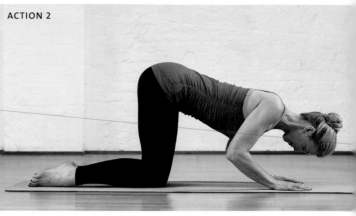

BOX PUSH UPS (LEVEL 3)

Adding Pilates principles maximizes the effectiveness of this popular gym exercise.

STARTING POSITION
Four-point Kneeling (page 54).

ACTION
1 Breathe in to prepare.
2 Breathe out and bend your elbows directly backward as you lower your upper body toward the mat in one long straight line.
3 Breathe in and hold the position.
4 Breathe out and slowly straighten your elbows to bring your trunk back to the Starting Position.
5 Repeat up to 10 times.

ONE ARM BOX PUSH UPS (LEVEL 4)

This adds the challenge of staying square and not rotating the trunk.

Start in Three-point Kneeling (page 55) and follow all the Action Points for Box Push Ups, repeating 5 times with each arm.

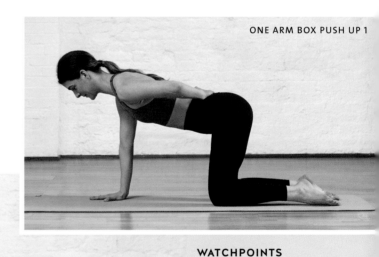

ONE ARM BOX PUSH UP 1

ONE ARM BOX PUSH UP 2

WATCHPOINTS

→ Use appropriate core connection to control your alignment and movements.

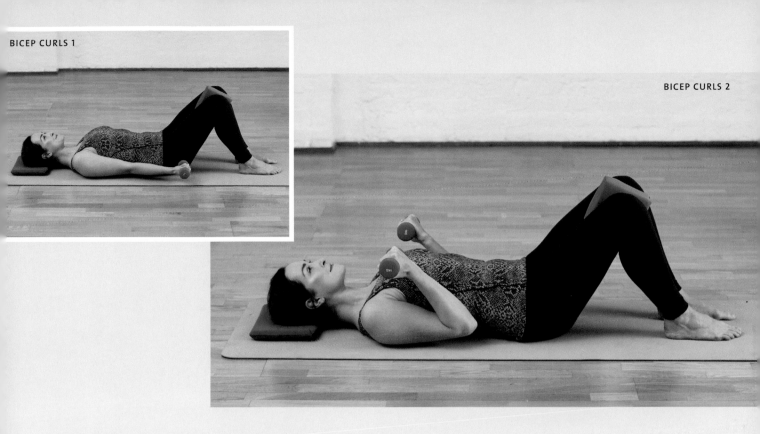

BICEP CURLS 1

ARM WEIGHTS SEQUENCE

BICEP CURLS, CHEST PRESSES, BACKSTROKE ARMS, FLIES (LEVEL 2)

This sequence of movements targets all the upper arm, shoulder and chest muscles in turn. We couldn't resist adding an optional bit of inner thigh work too. You will need a small cushion to squeeze and two light handweights. Start at no more than 0.5kg (1.1lb), gradually increasing if you can maintain good technique in all four movements. Be particularly cautious not to use too heavy a weight with Backstroke Arms (page 152).

STARTING POSITION

Relaxation Position (page 48) with hands by your sides, holding the weights, palms facing upward. Place a small cushion between your thighs and gently squeeze it. Maintain this inner-thigh squeeze throughout the sequence.

ACTION: BICEP CURLS

1 Breathe in to prepare and lengthen and lift both arms slightly from the mat.
2 Breathe out and bend both elbows toward your shoulders. Hover your upper arms above the mat.
3 Repeat 5 Bicep Curls.

WATCHPOINTS

→ Use appropriate core connection to control your alignment and movements.

→ Stay in control of your shoulders; keep them stable.

→ Make sure your collarbones remain open throughout.

→ Do fewer repetitions or use lighter weights if your technique starts to suffer.

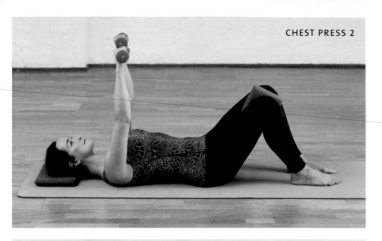

CHEST PRESS 2

ACTION: CHEST PRESSES

1 Breathe in and turn your palms to face away from you.
2 Breathe out and bring both hands up, shoulders stable, keeping wide across your collarbones and shoulders (think of Double Shoulder Drops, page 78).
3 Breathe in and bend your elbows out to the side in line with your shoulders.
4 Breathe out and press both arms up.
5 Breathe in and open the elbows to the side (but don't touch the mat).
6 Repeat 5 times.

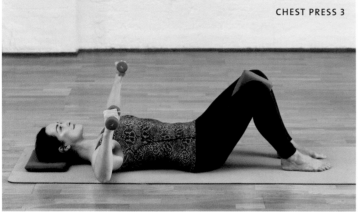

CHEST PRESS 3

ACTION: BACKSTROKE ARMS

1 When you've completed the presses bring your arms back up into Shoulder Drop position (page 78), palms facing away from you,
2 Breathe out and take one arm back toward the floor, the other hand down by your side toward the mat.
3 Breathe in and simultaneously bring both arms back to where you started. Repeat 5 times.

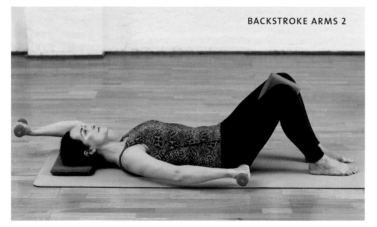

BACKSTROKE ARMS 2

ACTION: FLIES

1 Pause a moment to turn your palms to face inward.
2 Then breathe in and open both arms out to the side in a Fly action, elbows slightly bent and arms curved.
3 Breathe out and bring the arms back up again.
4 Repeat 5 times.
5 Finally, return to the Starting Position, arms back down by your side, palms facing up, ready to start the whole sequence again. Repeat the sequence twice.

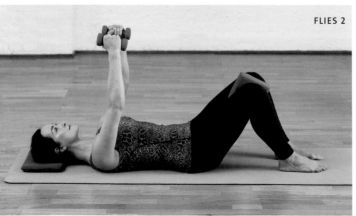

FLIES 2

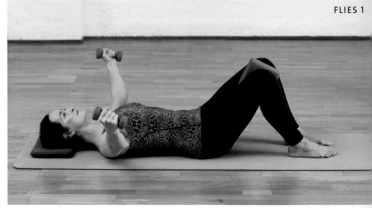

FLIES 1

STARTING POSITION

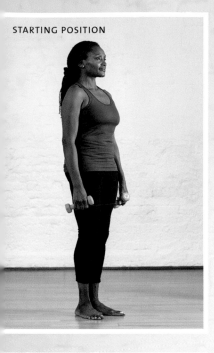

ACTION 1

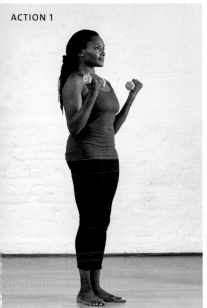

WATCHPOINTS

→ Use appropriate core connection to control your alignment and movements.

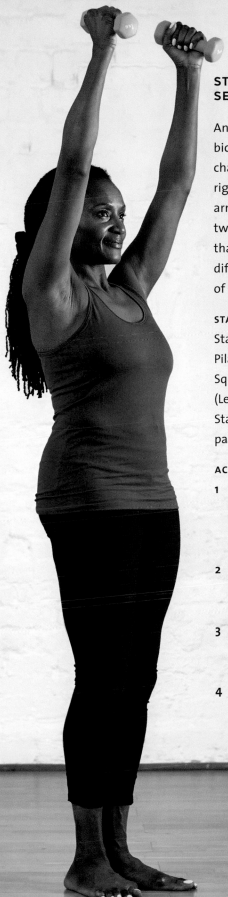

STANDING HAND WEIGHTS SEQUENCE (LEVEL 3)

Another sequence for you. This works the biceps, triceps and shoulder muscles. The change in hand position can be tricky to get right at first, but persevere to target different arm and shoulder muscles. You will need two light hand weights – start at no more than 0.5kg (1.1lb) – to lift overhead. Note: The different starting positions change the level of difficulty.

STARTING POSITION

Standing in Parallel (Level 3 – page 58), Pilates Stance (Level 3 – page 60), Pilates Squat (Level 4 – page 154) or Static Lunge (Level 5 – page 155, remember to swap legs). Start by holding the weights by your sides, palms facing inward.

ACTION: BICEPS PRESS

1 Breathe in and bend the elbows, turning your palms to face inward as you bring the weights toward your shoulders in a Bicep Curl.
2 Breathe out as you straighten both arms overhead, turning the palms to face each other.
3 Breathe in and bend your elbows again as you lower the arms back down to your shoulders, palms facing you again.
4 Breathe out as you straighten and lower your arms by your sides to return to the Starting Position.

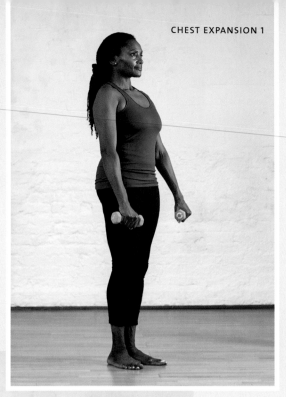

CHEST EXPANSION 1

ACTION: CHEST EXPANSION

1 Pause a moment before turning your palms to face backward.
2 Breathe in as you press back, taking the arms as far as you can behind you without disturbing your spine.
3 Still inhaling, turn your head left, pass through centre, and turn your head right.
4 Breathe out as you return your head to centre, then lengthen the arms forward, returning the arms to your sides.
5 Repeat the whole Biceps Press and Chest Expansion sequence 5 times, turning your head in a different way first each time. In a Static Lunge position, do 2 repetitions, then swap legs.

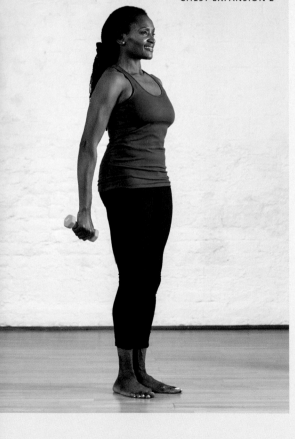

CHEST EXPANSION 2

WATCHPOINTS

→ Use appropriate core connection to control your alignment and movements.

→ Keep your feet grounded throughout, all toes in contact with the floor.

→ Control your shoulder stability and stay wide and open across your collarbones.

→ In Chest Expansion take a deep breath in (hence the name) and make that breath last until you've completed the neck turns.

→ Do not sway as you take the arms back or overhead.

SQUAT WITH HAND WEIGHTS SEQUENCE (LEVEL 4)

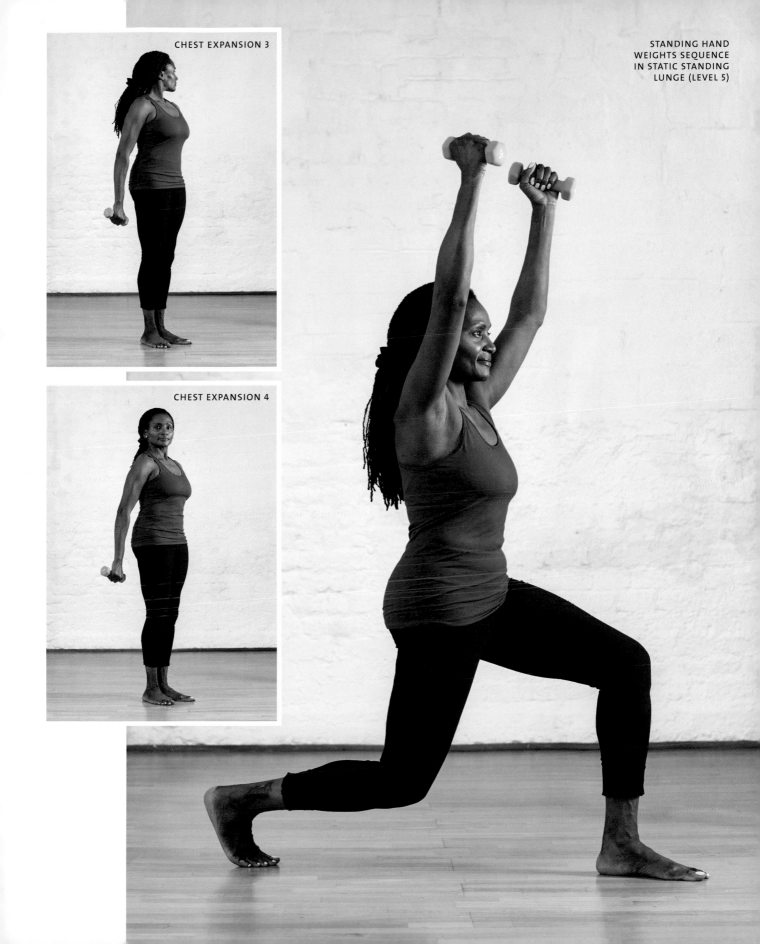

CHEST EXPANSION 3

CHEST EXPANSION 4

STANDING HAND
WEIGHTS SEQUENCE
IN STATIC STANDING
LUNGE (LEVEL 5)

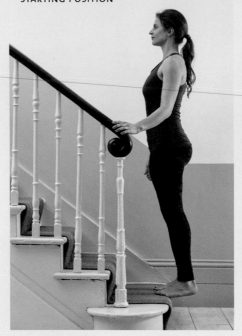

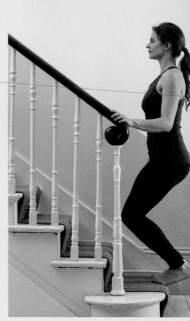

Buttocks & legs

No shape-up book would be complete without a section on buttocks and thighs – it's where women naturally store extra fat as part of our hormonal make-up. But that doesn't mean we have to be flabby! We'd all like round, toned buttocks and shapely legs. Do these exercises regularly and you will be on track.

THE LEG SHAPER (LEVEL 1)

We've put this exercise here to warm up your legs, especially the calves and ankles, in readiness for the exercises to come. A bottom step is helpful, but not essential, to add extra stretch. If working on a stair, hold the rail as you practise.

ACTION 3

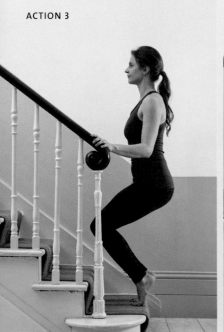

ACTION 4

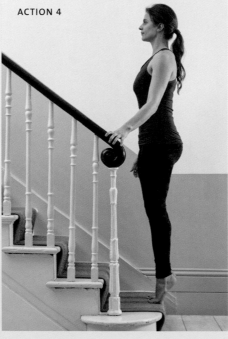

STARTING POSITION

Stand tall, feet in parallel. If using a step, keep your toes and the balls of both feet firmly planted on the step, with the back of your feet hovering just off the step. Hold the rail.

ACTION

1 Breathe in and lengthen up through the crown of the head.
2 Breathe out and bend both knees, sending them directly forward and folding at the hips and knees.
3 Breathe in and, with knees remaining bent, roll through the feet to lift the heels.
4 Breathe out and straighten both legs, keeping the heels lifted.
5 Breathe in and lower both heels, still lengthening up through the crown of your head. If on a step, lower your heels over the edge to give your calves an extra stretch.
6 Repeat the sequence up to 10 times.

ACTION 5

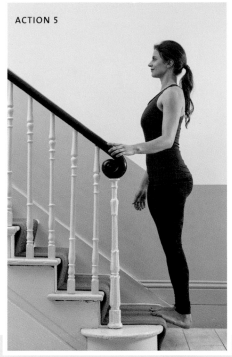

WALKING ON THE SPOT ON A STEP (LEVEL 1)

Another ankle and calf worker, which is similar to walking footwork on the Studio Universal Reformer.

STARTING POSITION
As for Leg Shaper.

ACTION
1 Breathing normally throughout, lift both heels, then bend one knee sending it directly forward, simultaneously lower the opposite heel down to give it a stretch.
2 Then transfer your weight swapping legs, all the while thinking of sending the crown of your head up, up, up. Both sides of your waist remain long. No wiggling!

ADD A DOUBLE FLOATING ARM (LEVEL 4)

If you are not working on stairs, add an arm raise when high on your toes – this challenges your balance.

WALKING ON THE
SPOT ON A STEP

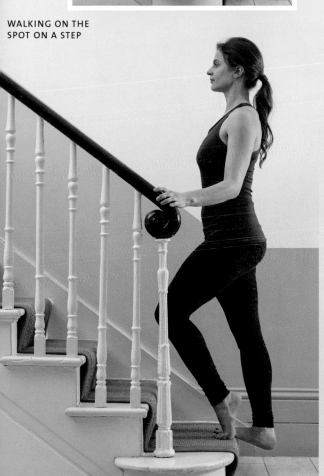

WATCHPOINTS
➔ Use appropriate core connection to control your alignment and movements.

➔ Think of your three body weights – head, ribcage, pelvis – and keep them in a line. Do not stick your bottom out or tuck your tailbone under.

➔ Ensure your knees or ankles do not roll in or out.

➔ To help alignment, think of pulling up through the inner ankle bone, then the insides of your knees and thighs, right up through the spine and the top of your head.

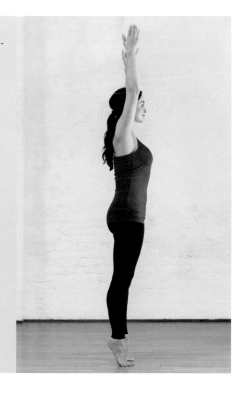

BRIDGE SERIES

BASIC BRIDGE (LEVEL 2)

Bridges are brilliant buttock toning exercises – and of course we couldn't resist adding a few new twists to challenge you more.

STARTING POSITION

Relaxation Position (page 48), preferably without a pillow or towel under your head. If more comfortable with a pillow, choose a flat one.

ACTION

1 Breathe in to prepare.
2 Breathe out as you send your knees away from you and lift your bottom from the mat, raising your spine in one movement until you end up in a long diagonal line.
3 Breathe in and hold the position.
4 Breathe out and lower the spine in one piece.
5 Repeat up to 10 times.

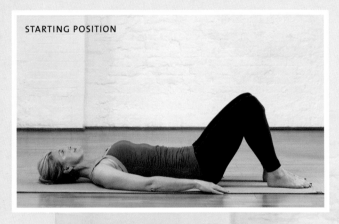

STARTING POSITION

WATCHPOINTS

➔ Use appropriate core connection to control your alignment and movements.

➔ Do not be tempted to curl the spine; let it move as one.

➔ Send your knees away as you lift your hips.

➔ Keep the weight even on both feet.

➔ Take care not to bridge too high.

➔ Pelvis must stay level, both sides of the chest long.

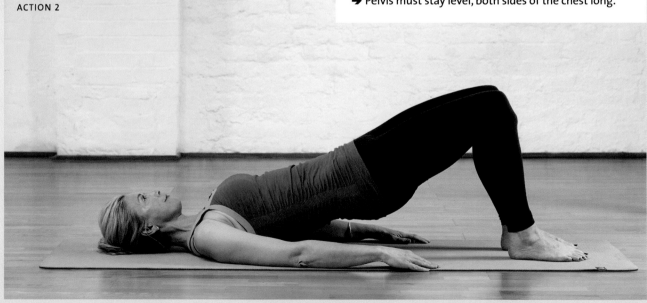

ACTION 2

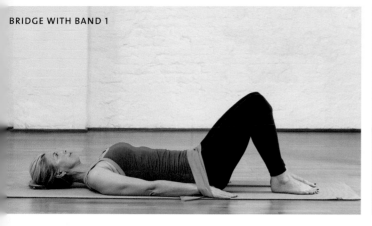

BRIDGE WITH BAND 1

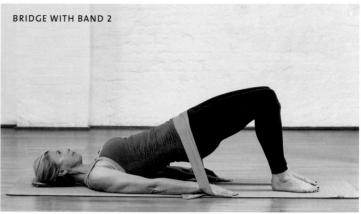

BRIDGE WITH BAND 2

BRIDGE WITH BAND (LEVEL 3)

The band adds resistance to the movement, making your muscles work harder. Check the band provides enough slack/give that you can bridge up, but retains enough resistance to make your buttocks work harder.

Wrap the band around your hands and hold in place with your thumbs. Try first with the hands on the mat... for more challenge, have them hovering just off the mat!

Then follow all the directions for Basic Bridge, opposite.

BRIDGE AND LEG EXTENSION (LEVEL 4)

At the height of the Bridge, straighten one leg. Then bend the knee again, before repeating with the other leg. Add extra breaths as needed. Repeat up to 3 times with each leg before lowering. (Pelvis must stay level.)

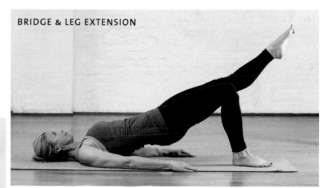

BRIDGE & LEG EXTENSION

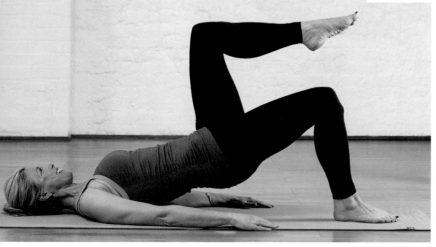

BRIDGE & KNEE FOLD

BRIDGE AND KNEE FOLD (LEVEL 4)

The Knee Fold increases the challenge to your core dramatically. Keep your pelvis level and lifted and feel your buttocks and waist working. Return your foot to the floor before coming down.

BRIDGE ON TOES (LEVELS 3 AND 4)

For Level 3, bridge up, then lift your heels to rise onto your toes. Lower your heels before coming down.

For Level 4, rise onto your toes before bridging up and stay on your toes until you go back down again.

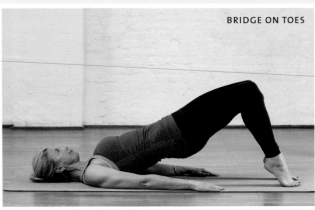

BRIDGE ON TOES

BRIDGE ON TOES WITH BAND

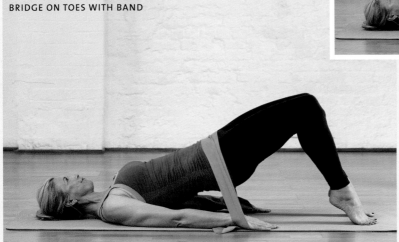

PRETZEL BRIDGE (LEVEL 4)

To target the glutes even more, from the Starting Position, bend one knee and place the ankle just above the other knee. Keep the pelvis square before bridging up. This stretches the "pretzel" side and strengthens the supporting side. Add a band for extra challenge.

PRETZEL BRIDGE A

PRETZEL BRIDGE B

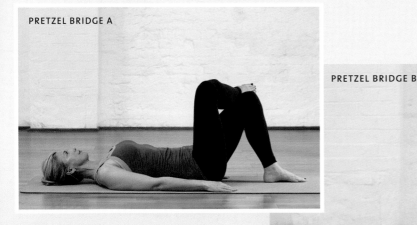

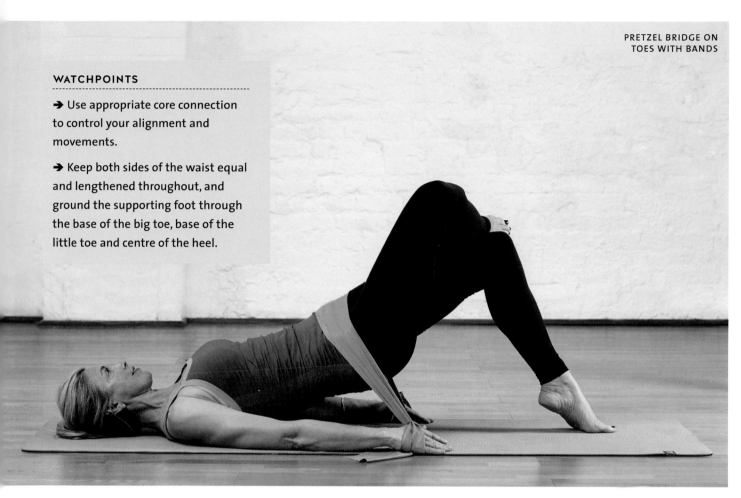

WATCHPOINTS

→ Use appropriate core connection
to control your alignment and
movements.

→ Keep both sides of the waist equal
and lengthened throughout, and
ground the supporting foot through
the base of the big toe, base of the
little toe and centre of the heel.

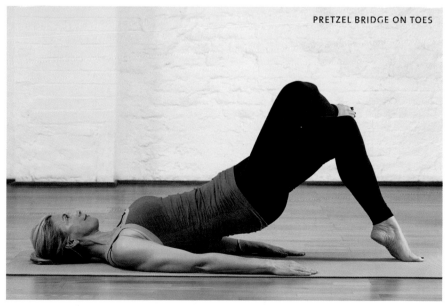

PRETZEL BRIDGE ON TOES
(LEVEL 5)

Just when you thought it couldn't get
any tougher... follow all the directions for
Pretzel Bridge, but rise onto your toes at
the height of the Bridge. Then when you
feel ready, come onto your toes before
bridging up.

LEG PULL BACK SERIES

BACK BRIDGE (LEVEL 3)

The Leg Pull Back series of exercises works you top to toe. It was tough deciding whether to place these exercises in the arm or buttock section of the book, because they work both areas.

    We start the series with Back Bridge, which prepares you for Leg Pull Back Prep (page 166).

STARTING POSITION
Sit tall on the mat with knees bent in front of you, hip-width apart, feet flat on the floor. Place your hands by your sides in line with your shoulders, palms flat on the mat, fingers facing forward. Depending on the length of your arms and body, you may need to bend your elbows slightly. Ensure that you are in a lengthened position and your shoulders are open.

ACTION
1 Breathe in to prepare.
2 Breathe out and lift your bottom from the mat, sending your hips to the ceiling and knees forward.
3 Breathe in and hold this position.
4 Breathe out and lower with control.
5 Repeat up to 10 times.

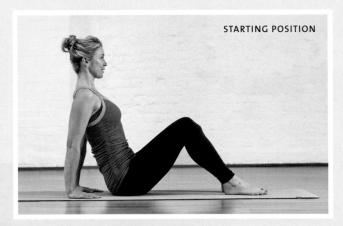
STARTING POSITION

ACTION 2

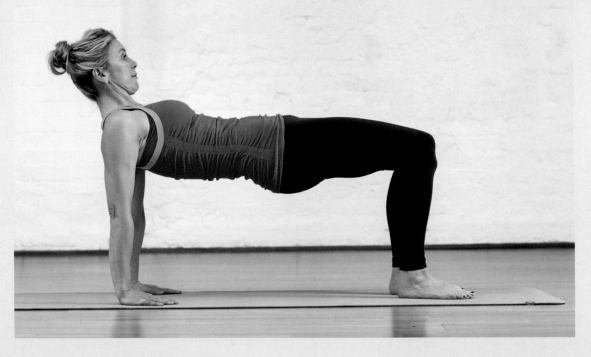

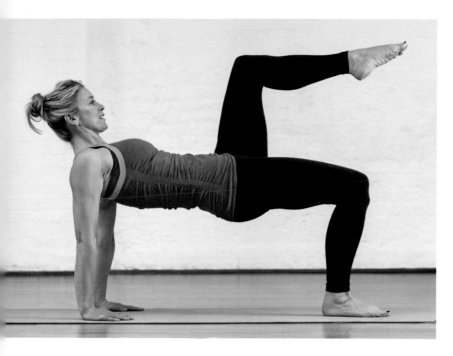

BACK BRIDGE AND KNEE FOLD (LEVEL 4)

Fold one knee up at the height of the Back Bridge (opposite). Return the foot before bridging down. Remain central. Repeat 3 times with each leg before lowering down. You can also stay up in a bridge as you swap legs.

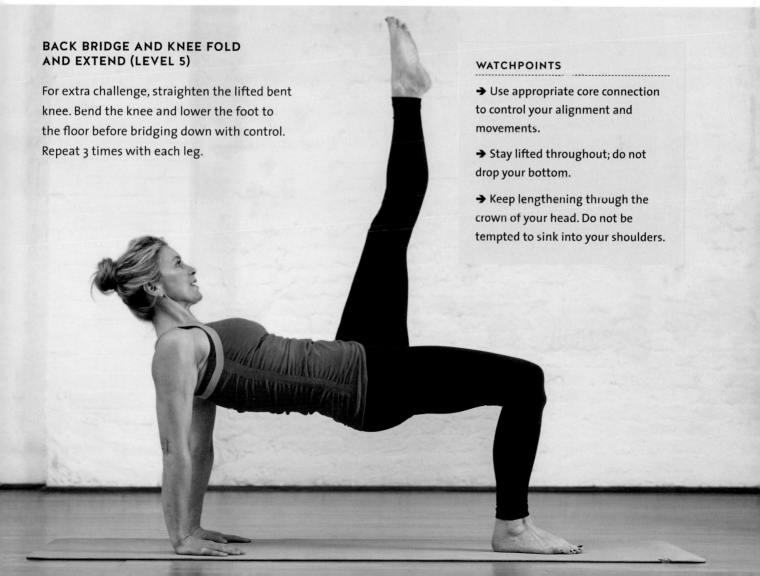

BACK BRIDGE AND KNEE FOLD AND EXTEND (LEVEL 5)

For extra challenge, straighten the lifted bent knee. Bend the knee and lower the foot to the floor before bridging down with control. Repeat 3 times with each leg.

WATCHPOINTS

→ Use appropriate core connection to control your alignment and movements.

→ Stay lifted throughout; do not drop your bottom.

→ Keep lengthening through the crown of your head. Do not be tempted to sink into your shoulders.

BACK BRIDGE, KNEE FOLD, EXTEND, AND LOWER (LEVEL 6)

For extra challenge, lower the straight leg to the floor as low as you can go without disturbing the pelvis. Fold the knee in and lower the foot before repeating with the other leg. Repeat 3 times to each side before lowering your bottom onto the mat.

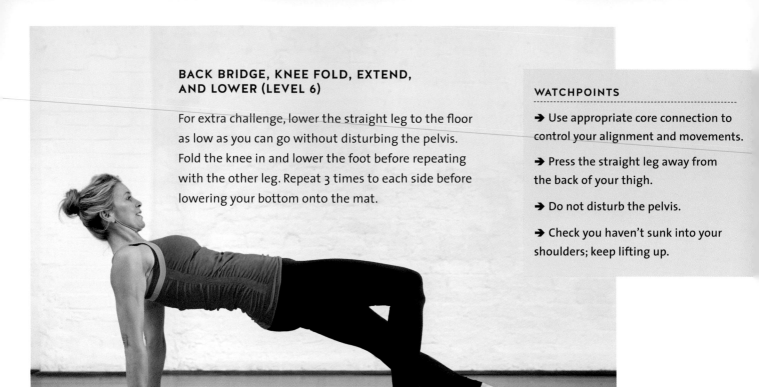

PRETZEL BACK BRIDGE (LEVEL 5)

This version really targets the deep buttock muscles. The supporting side gets toned, while the "pretzel" side gets a stretch.

STARTING POSITION
As for Back Bridge (page 162), but bend one knee and place the ankle across just above the knee. Keep the pelvis square.

ACTION
1 Breathe in to prepare.
2 Breathe out and bridge up.
3 Breathe in and come back down to the Starting Position.
4 Repeat 5 times with each leg.

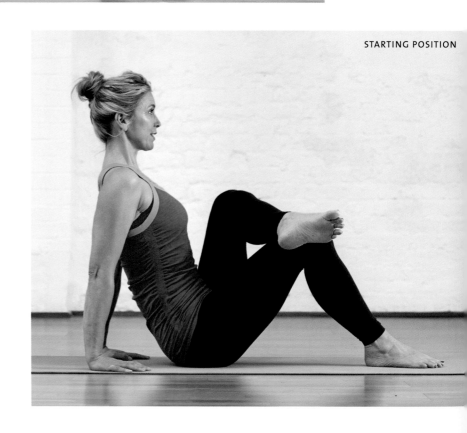

STARTING POSITION

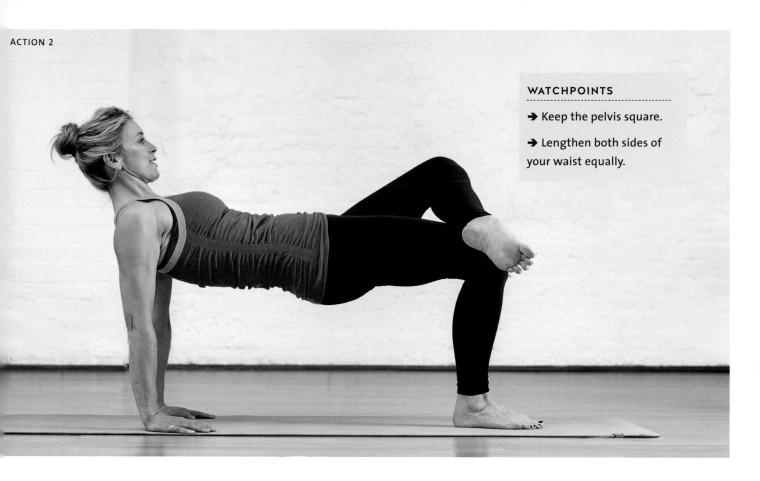

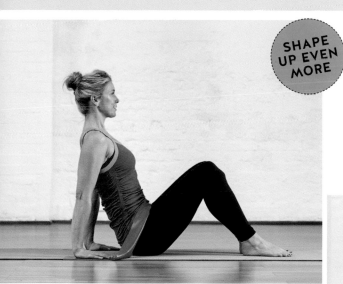

SHAPE UP EVEN MORE

ADDING RESISTANCE WITH A STRETCH BAND

You can practise all versions of Back Bridge with a stretch band wrapped around your pelvis to make your buttocks work harder and increase the toning potential. Hold the ends with your hands, making sure there is enough give in the band to lift up against. The band should offer resistance but not restrict you.

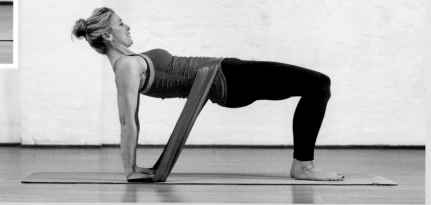

LEG PULL BACK PREP (LEVEL 5)

A challenging exercise, this requires a great deal of control and strength in the upper body to maintain a stable torso while mobilizing the hips, both strengthening and lengthening the surrounding muscles. Back Bridge (page 162) will have prepared you.

STARTING POSITION

Sit tall, legs lengthened out in front of you, inner thighs connected and feet softly pointed. Place your hands behind you, palms flat, fingers facing toward you.

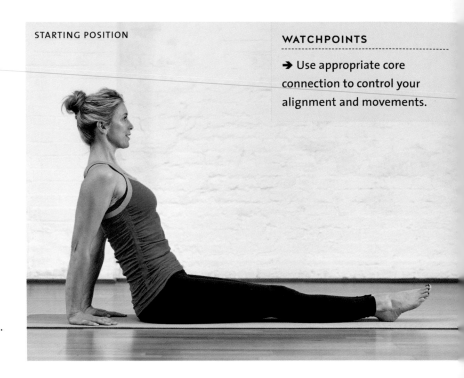

→ Use appropriate core connection to control your alignment and movements.

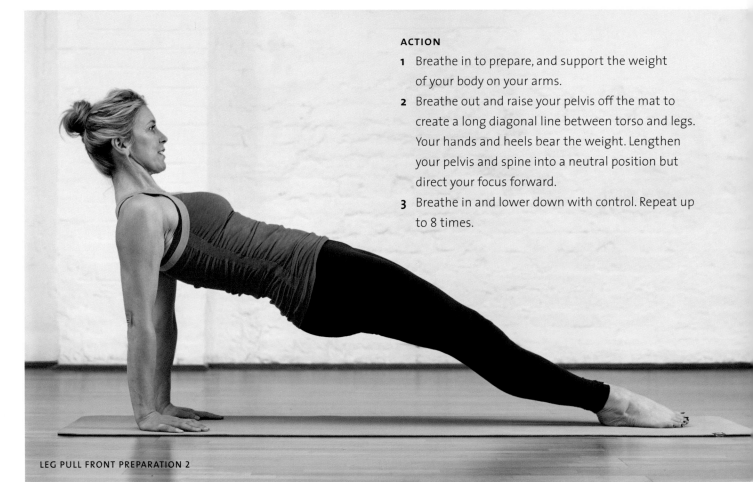

ACTION

1 Breathe in to prepare, and support the weight of your body on your arms.
2 Breathe out and raise your pelvis off the mat to create a long diagonal line between torso and legs. Your hands and heels bear the weight. Lengthen your pelvis and spine into a neutral position but direct your focus forward.
3 Breathe in and lower down with control. Repeat up to 8 times.

LEG PULL FRONT PREPARATION 2

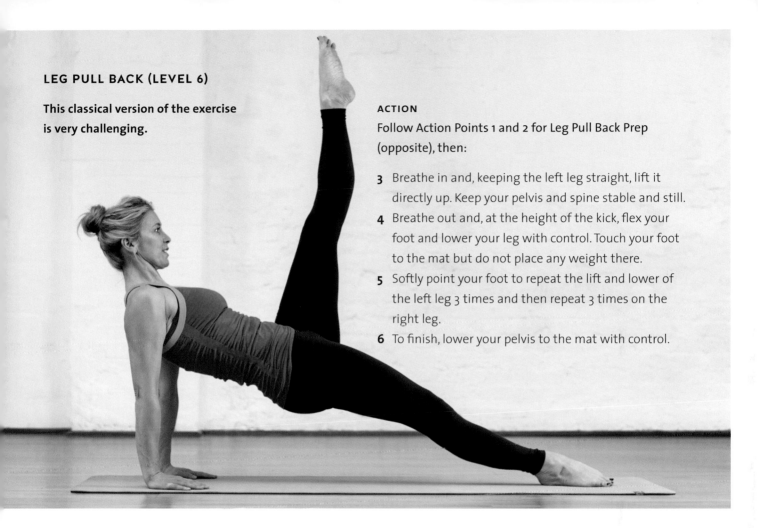

LEG PULL BACK (LEVEL 6)

This classical version of the exercise is very challenging.

ACTION

Follow Action Points 1 and 2 for Leg Pull Back Prep (opposite), then:

3 Breathe in and, keeping the left leg straight, lift it directly up. Keep your pelvis and spine stable and still.

4 Breathe out and, at the height of the kick, flex your foot and lower your leg with control. Touch your foot to the mat but do not place any weight there.

5 Softly point your foot to repeat the lift and lower of the left leg 3 times and then repeat 3 times on the right leg.

6 To finish, lower your pelvis to the mat with control.

WATCHPOINTS

➡ Keep your pelvis square and stable and spine lengthened.

➡ Move your legs independently of your pelvis and spine.

➡ Lift the weight of your body away from your arms and keep the front of your shoulders and your chest open.

➡ Keep your neck lengthened and your focus directly forward.

➡ Lengthen both arms and legs fully throughout, but do not lock your elbows or knees.

LEG PULL BACK

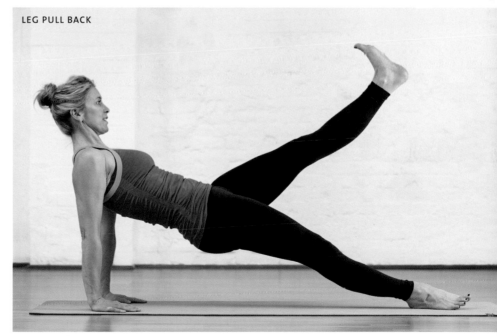

PILATES SQUAT SERIES

PILATES SQUAT (LEVEL 1)

The Pilates Squat is a useful exercise for working the buttocks and legs and adds a gentle cardio element to your workout. We've got some fun variations, including with weights, start with 0.5kg (1.1lb), or a long, light stretch band.

STARTING POSITION
Stand tall on the floor (not your mat) arms lengthened by your sides, palms facing inward.

ACTION

1 Breathe in and bend your hips, knees and ankles into a small squat. You will naturally hinge forward from your hips, but keep your spine straight. Reach your arms forward to help you balance.

2 Breathe out and press the floor away as you straighten up and stand tall.

3 Repeat up to 10 times.

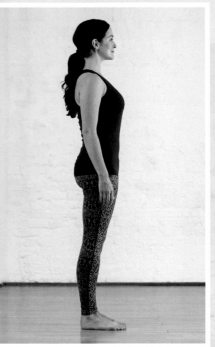

PILATES SQUAT 2

WATCHPOINTS

→ Use appropriate core connection to control your alignment and movements.

→ Don't squat too low – avoid taking your bottom lower than knee-level.

→ Check that your knees and ankles do not roll in or out.

→ Place equal weight between your left and right leg.

→ Keep all your toes on the floor.

→ For the simple Squat your heels stay down.

→ Keep your pelvis and spine in neutral.

SQUATS WITH HEEL RAISE (LEVEL 2)

This adds an extra challenge to your alignment and works the calves!

Rise onto your toes in the Squat. Lower your heels before returning to upright. Repeat up to 10 times.

ADD A STRETCH BAND FOR EXTRA GLUTEAL WORK (LEVEL 2)

Wrap a stretch band around the bottom of your bottom/top of your thighs and hold the ends in each hand before squatting. This intensifies the work of the gluteal muscles.

WITH HEEL RAISE

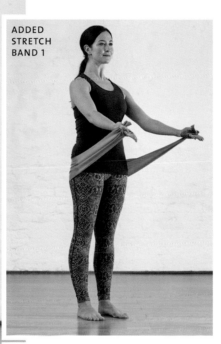

ADDED STRETCH BAND 1

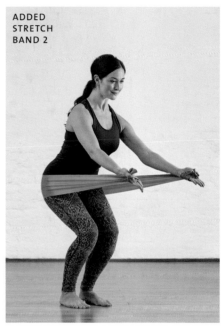

ADDED STRETCH BAND 2

ADD WEIGHTS AND BICEP CURLS (LEVEL 3)

Start holding weights or stand on a long, light stretch band holding the ends.

Do 3 Bicep Curls (page 134) when you are in the Squat before returning to upright. Alternatively, Bicep Curl as you squat!

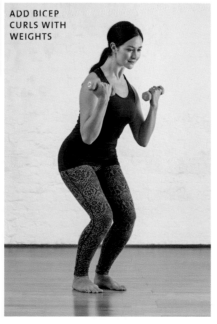

ADD BICEP CURLS WITH WEIGHTS

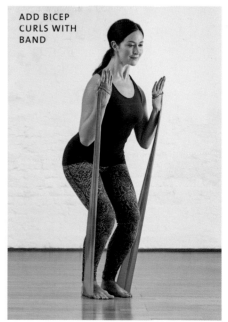

ADD BICEP CURLS WITH BAND

DYNAMIC LUNGES

Applying Pilates principles to this common gym exercise makes it even more effective. It is a multi-toner, giving your gluteals, thighs and calves a great workout. Like Squats, it adds a gentle cardio element to your workout, especially when you add an arm action.

It is easier to maintain good alignment with a Backward Lunge, so if you are new to Lunges start backwards... the end result will be the same position so you won't see a difference in the photos.

DYNAMIC BACKWARD LUNGE (LEVEL 1)

STARTING POSITION
Stand tall, feet hip-width apart and in parallel (page 58). Double-check that your pelvis and spine are in neutral.

STARTING POSITION

ACTION
1 Breathe in as you step backward with your right foot, bending the right knee, your back heel lifts. As you do this, your front knee will simultaneously bend; you are aiming for a right angle, the ankle should be directly beneath the knee. Try to stay as upright as possible.
2 Breathe out as you straighten up and step back to the Starting Position.
3 Repeat up to 6 times with each leg.

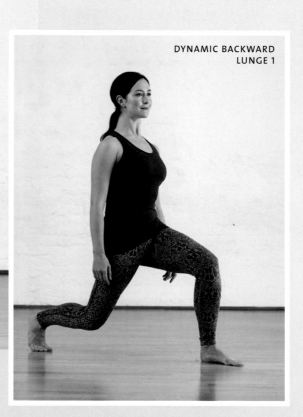

DYNAMIC BACKWARD LUNGE 1

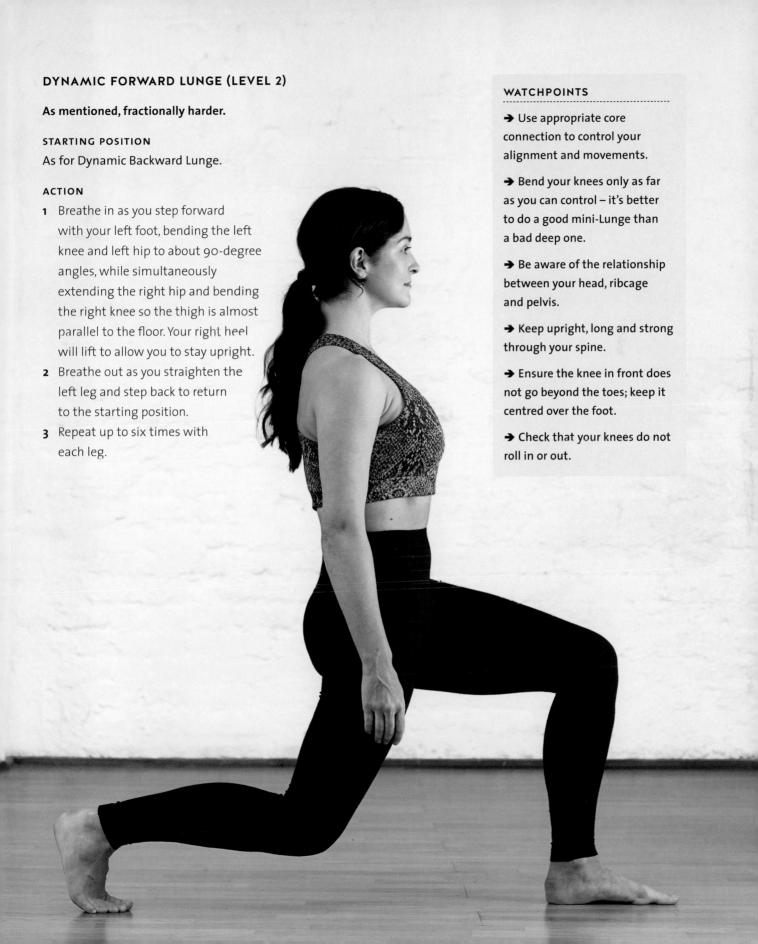

DYNAMIC FORWARD LUNGE (LEVEL 2)

As mentioned, fractionally harder.

STARTING POSITION
As for Dynamic Backward Lunge.

ACTION

1 Breathe in as you step forward with your left foot, bending the left knee and left hip to about 90-degree angles, while simultaneously extending the right hip and bending the right knee so the thigh is almost parallel to the floor. Your right heel will lift to allow you to stay upright.

2 Breathe out as you straighten the left leg and step back to return to the starting position.

3 Repeat up to six times with each leg.

WATCHPOINTS

→ Use appropriate core connection to control your alignment and movements.

→ Bend your knees only as far as you can control – it's better to do a good mini-Lunge than a bad deep one.

→ Be aware of the relationship between your head, ribcage and pelvis.

→ Keep upright, long and strong through your spine.

→ Ensure the knee in front does not go beyond the toes; keep it centred over the foot.

→ Check that your knees do not roll in or out.

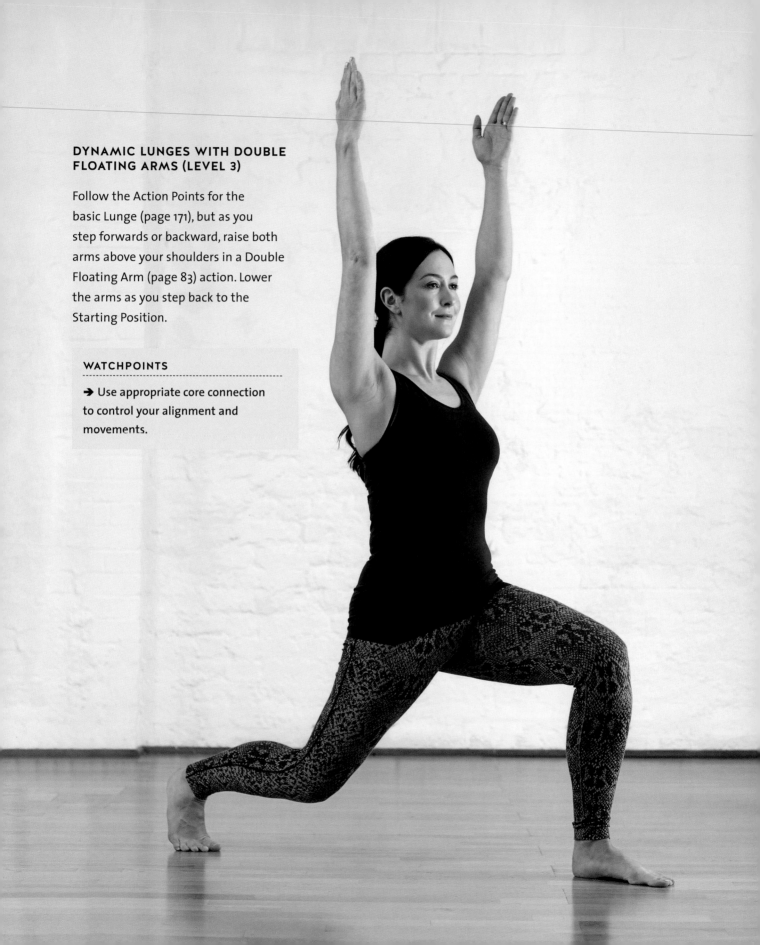

DYNAMIC LUNGES WITH DOUBLE FLOATING ARMS (LEVEL 3)

Follow the Action Points for the basic Lunge (page 171), but as you step forwards or backward, raise both arms above your shoulders in a Double Floating Arm (page 83) action. Lower the arms as you step back to the Starting Position.

WATCHPOINTS

➔ Use appropriate core connection to control your alignment and movements.

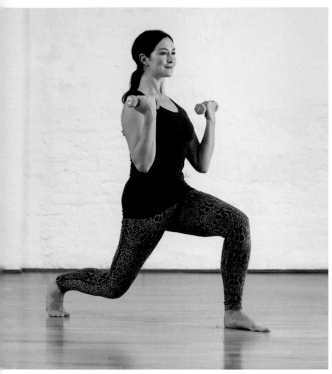

DYNAMIC LUNGES WITH BICEP CURLS (LEVEL 3)

Start with arms by your sides, palms facing inward. As you lunge backward or forward, bend your elbows in Bicep Curls (page 134), bringing your hands to your shoulders and turning the palms to face you.

DYNAMIC LUNGES WITH ARM CIRCLES (LEVEL 4)

After stepping backward or forward, circle your arms once before stepping back to repeat on the other leg.

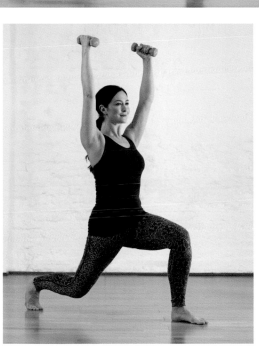

DYNAMIC LUNGES WITH DOUBLE FLOATING ARM WITH WEIGHTS (LEVEL 4)

To raise your heart rate even more, hold light hand weights as you lunge – no more than 0.5kg (1.1lb).

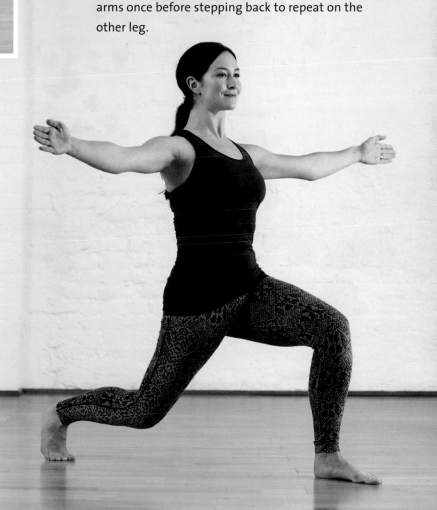

The back

Including back extension exercises in every workout is a must – they are probably the ultimate anti-gravity and thus anti-ageing exercises. Nothing is more unflattering than a slouched posture. To maintain an upright posture all day requires strong upper-back muscles, and that's the goal of these exercises. They also tone around your upper back and shoulder blades.

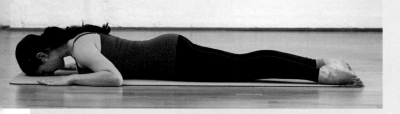

STARTING POSITION

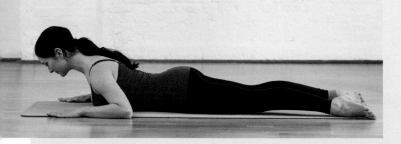

COBRA PREP ACTION 2

COBRA (AND OTHER REPTILES) SERIES

COBRA PREP (LEVEL 1)

From Cobra Prep to Full Cobra and variations, this series gets progressively more challenging but also progressively more rewarding.

STARTING POSITION

Prone (page 58), resting your forehead on the mat (on a folded towel, if necessary). Your legs are straight, slightly wider than hip-width apart and turned out from the hips. Bend your elbows and position your hands slightly wider than and above your shoulders, palms facing down. Make sure your shoulders are released and your collarbones wide.

ACTION

1 Breathe in to prepare.
2 Breathe out as you begin to lengthen the front of your neck to roll and lift your head and then your chest away from the mat. Keep your lower ribs in contact with the mat, open your chest and focus on directing it forward.
3 Breathe in as you hold this lengthened lifted position.
4 Breathe out as you return your chest and head sequentially to the mat.
5 Repeat up to 10 times.

WATCHPOINTS

→ Use core connection to support your lower back.

→ Keep your legs on the mat, reaching away from you throughout.

→ For Cobra Prep, keep your elbows down.

COBRA PREP WITH NECK TURN (LEVEL 1)

There is no added toning power in this exercise, but it feels wonderful to move your neck freely in this extended position.

ACTION
Follow Action Points 1 and 2 for Cobra Prep, then:

3 Breathe in and turn your head gently to one side.
4 Breathing out, turn your head back through centre and to the other side.
5 Breathe in, return your head to centre.
6 Breathe out and slowly lower down with control.

WATCHPOINTS
....

→ Use appropriate core connection to control your alignment and movements.

→ Grow, grow, grow – think forward and up.

→ Don't put too much pressure down into the arms; they are there to lightly support you, not press you up.

→ Think of your breastbone shining forward.

→ Return to the mat with length and control, do not collapse.

COBRA PREP WITH NECK TURN 3

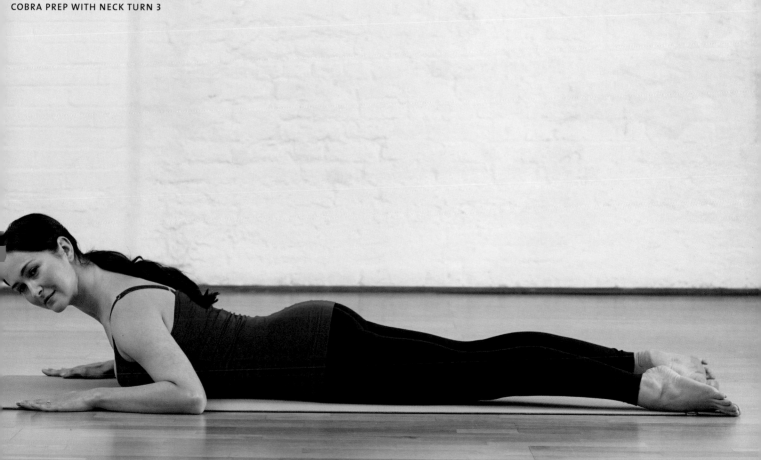

FULL COBRA (LEVEL 4)

Don't just think about the back of your body in this exercise – to do it well you need to lengthen the front of your body and give your lower back support from your core connection.

STARTING POSITION
As for Cobra Prep (page 174).

ACTION

1 Breathe in to prepare.

2 Breathe out as you lengthen the front of your neck to roll and lift your head, then continue to peel your body away from the mat. Lift the breastbone, then the ribcage, abdominal area and front of your pelvis. As the body wheels off the mat, your arms begin to straighten. Continue to lengthen your legs.

3 Breathe in and stay lengthened and lifted.

4 Breathe out as you lengthen the spine down, first the front of your pelvis, then the abdominal area, ribcage, breastbone and finally your head.

5 Repeat up to 8 times before coming up into Four-point Kneeling (page 54). Bring your feet together and fold back into Rest Position (page 108).

WATCHPOINTS

→ Use appropriate core connection to control your alignment and movements.

→ At the height of Full Cobra, allow your hips to open and the front of your pelvis to lose contact with the mat.

→ Your arms may not fully straighten, depending on the length of your spine and arms, and your flexibility.

→ Keep your legs on the mat, reaching away from you.

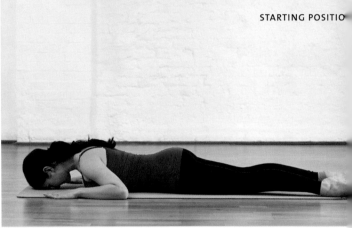

STARTING POSITIO

FULL COBRA 2

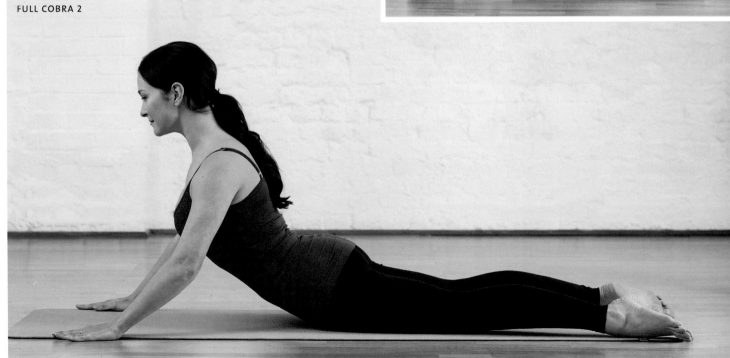

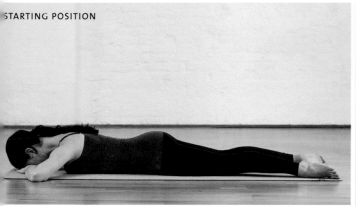

➔ Do not disturb your pelvis when lifting or beating your legs.

➔ Let the opening and closing action of the legs come from your hips.

➔ Keep the opening of the legs small.

➔ Maintain the slight turn-out of your legs from the hips.

PRONE BEATS 2

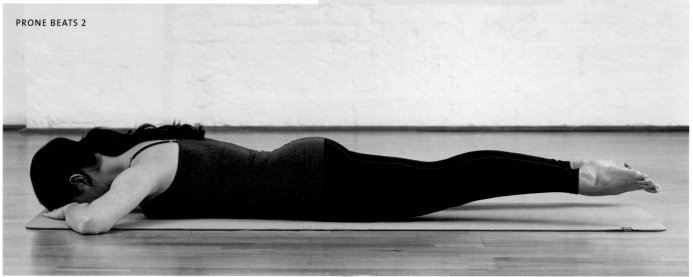

PRONE BEATS (LEVEL 4)

This is really, really good for working your buttocks and inner thighs.

STARTING POSITION

Prone (page 58), with legs straight and inner thighs connected and turned out from the hips. Rest your forehead on the backs of your hands.

ACTION

1 Breathe in to prepare.
2 Breathe out as you lengthen and lift both legs slightly away from the mat.
3 Breathe in for a count of 5 as you open and close your inner thighs, beating them briskly together 5 times. The accent is "in", "in".
4 Breathe out for another count of 5 as you repeat the brisk beating action.
5 Repeat up to 3 times.

LIZARD (LEVEL 3)

This Cobra variation brings a rotation element to the extension. We've added another version with a knee bend and ankle articulation to keep you well coordinated. Pilates aficionados will recognize the origin of the leg action.

STARTING POSITION

Prone (page 58), resting your forehead on the mat or a folded towel. Your legs are straight, shoulder-width apart and slightly turned out from the hips. Bend your elbows and position your hands slightly wider than and above your shoulders, palms facing down. Release your shoulders and widen your collarbones.

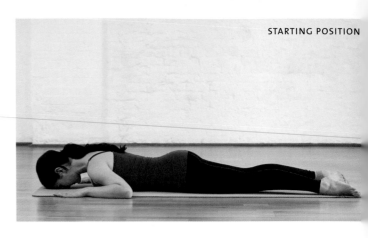

ACTION

1 Breathe in as you lengthen the front of the neck to roll and lift your head, then your neck until they are in line with your spine.

2 Breathe out as you open your left shoulder by pressing gently on your left hand, rotating your head, spine and ribs to the left until you are looking over your left shoulder.

3 Breathe into that open rib and hold the position.

4 Breathe out and slowly return to the Starting Position, moving through your ribs, shoulders and finally bringing your head back to rest.

5 Repeat on the right side, then repeat the sequence up 8 times.

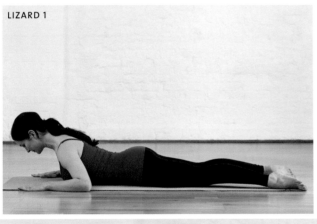

LIZARD 1

WATCHPOINTS

➔ Use appropriate core connection to control your alignment and movements.

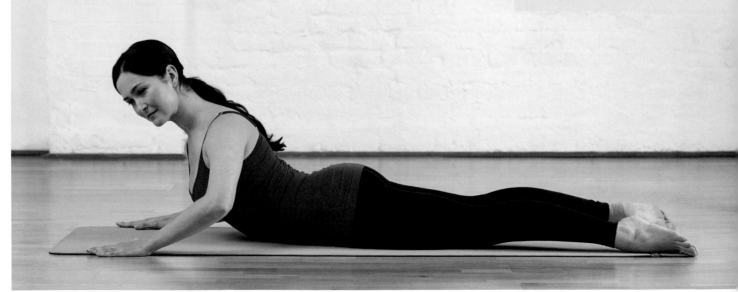

LIZARD 2

LIZARD WITH LEGS (LEVEL 3)

Add the leg and ankle action to mobilize your knees and ankles and gently lengthen the front of your thighs.

ACTION
Follow Action Points 1 and 2 for Lizard (you are looking over your left shoulder), then:

3 Breathe in as you bend your right knee. Keep the knee on the mat.

4 Breathe out as you flex, point and flex your ankle in a small pulsing action.

5 Breathing in and pointing again, simultaneously straighten your right knee and sequentially return to the Starting Position.

6 Repeat on the other side, looking over your right shoulder and bending and flexing your left knee and ankle.

7 Repeat up to 4 times with each side. Experiment with the breathing pattern if it doesn't work for you.

WATCHPOINTS

➔ Keep your pelvis grounded and centred throughout the exercise.

➔ Press gently through your arm to help your upper body rotation, but don't push hard.

➔ Do not turn your head further than feels comfortable.

➔ Keep both collarbones wide and open.

➔ Control your return; do not collapse down.

➔ You may not be able to extend as high or twist as far as our model.

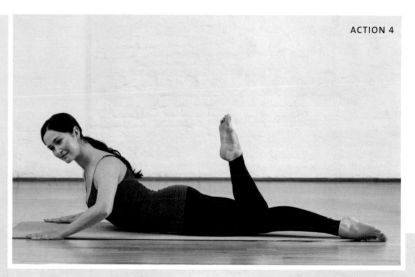

ACTION 4

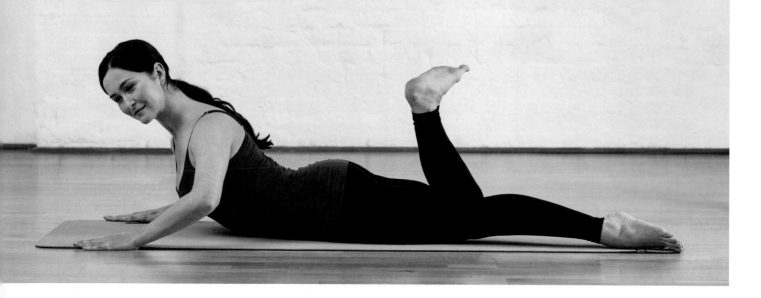

ACTION 4 WITH FLEX

DART (LEVEL 1)

This works on your back muscles as well as your inner thighs and gluteals.
There is a lot happening at once with this exercise, so read through several
times before trying it. You can also practise with legs slightly wider than
hip-width apart and turned out from the hips.

WATCHPOINTS

→ Use appropriate core connection to control your
alignment and movements.

→ Take care not to tip your head back too far;
keep your gaze down throughout.

→ Follow the right order of events: first the head
lifts, then the neck and, once they are in line with
the upper spine, the upper spine extends.

→ Keep your ribs connected down into your waist.

→ Do not be tempted to lift your legs; keep
them grounded.

STARTING POSITION

Prone (page 58), with a folded towel or flat cushion
beneath your forehead (if needed). Lengthen your arms
by the side of your body, resting on the mat, palms facing
upward. Lengthen your legs, base of the big toes touching.

ACTION

1 Breathe in to prepare.
2 Breathe out as you start to extend the upper spine,
  lengthening and lifting first your head, then your
  neck, then your upper spine one vertebra at a time.
  Simultaneously draw your legs together, connecting
  the inner thighs to bring them into a parallel
  position. At the same time, lengthen your arms away
  from you and lift them slightly as they turn outward
  so the palms now face the body.
3 Breathe in and maintain this lengthened position.
4 Breathe out as you sequentially return the
  upper back, then the neck, then head to the mat,
  simultaneously relaxing your legs and turning your
  arms back to the Starting Position.
5 Repeat up to 10 times.

STARTING POSITION

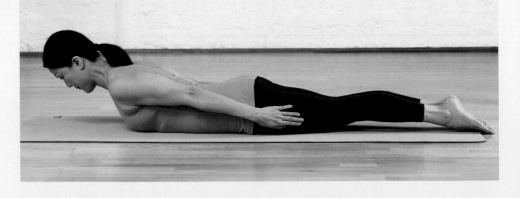

ACTION 2

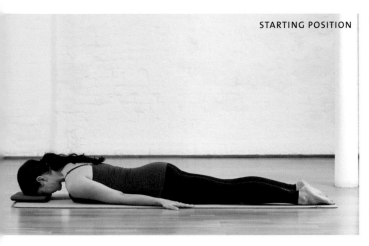

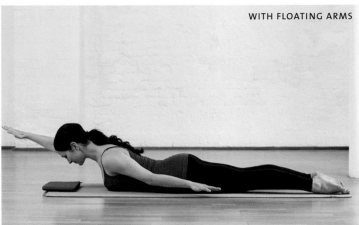

DART WITH ONE FLOATING ARM (LEVEL 3)

Here we up the challenge by adding an arm action – this is two levels up because the arms exert a lot more load. I like to imagine I'm in a swimming pool when practising. As the arm presses back down it's like pushing through water. Notice how you have to change palm position. This may look difficult but feels natural.

STARTING POSITION
As for Dart, but palms down.

ACTION
Follow Action Points 1 and 2 for Dart, then:

3 Breathe in and float one arm up, out to the side and above you. Keep the arm away from the ground at shoulder level as it moves. Turn your arm naturally as it floats up.

4 Breathe out and turn your palm to face away from you, then press the arm back down by your side. Maintain your back extension – if anything, feel it increase as you press the arm away.

5 Repeat twice, alternating arms, before slowly returning to the Starting Position sequentially and with control.

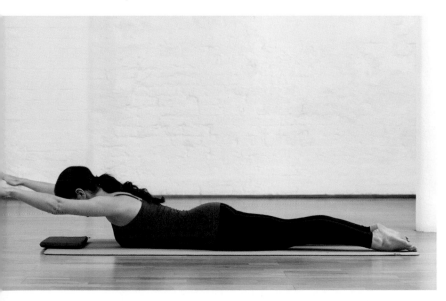

DART WITH TWO FLOATING ARMS (LEVEL 4)

Float both arms up one at a time when your back is extended for significantly more challenge. Return the arms to your side before you lower down.

DART WITH SIMULTANEOUS DOUBLE FLOATING ARMS (LEVEL 5)

Repeat as above, but floating both arms simultaneously.

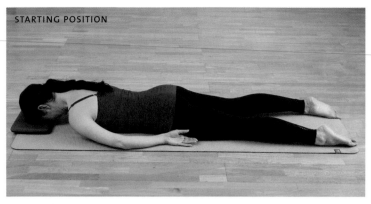

STARTING POSITION

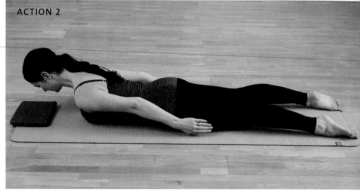

ACTION 2

DART WITH SIDE REACH (LEVEL 3)

These versions of the exercise work your back, shoulders and waist. It's a good idea to refresh your memory of Side Reach (page 104) before starting because you need to move sequentially in the same way.

STARTING POSITION

As for Dart (page 180) but with feet hip-width or, if more comfortable, shoulder-width apart.

ACTION

1 Breathe in to prepare.
2 Breathe out as you lengthen and lift first your head, then your neck, then your upper spine one vertebra at a time. At the same time lengthen your arms away and lift them slightly as they turn outward so the palms face your body.
3 Breathe in and hold the position.
4 Breathe out and leading with your head, neck and upper back, side-bend to the right. Keep your pelvis central and hover your breastbone just off the mat on one plane.
5 Breathe in as you lengthen up and side-bend back to centre.
6 Repeat twice to each side before lowering back to the Starting Position with control.

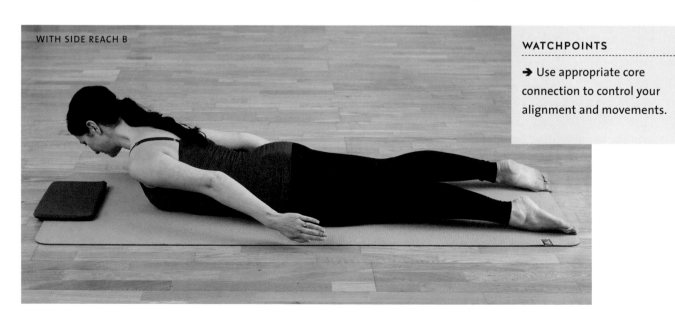

WITH SIDE REACH B

WATCHPOINTS

→ Use appropriate core connection to control your alignment and movements.

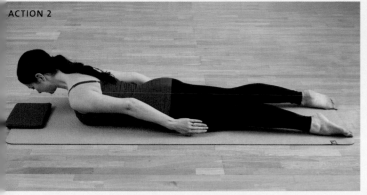

ACTION 2

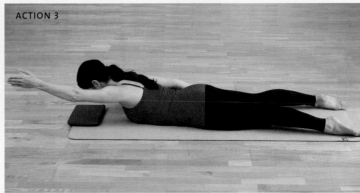

ACTION 3

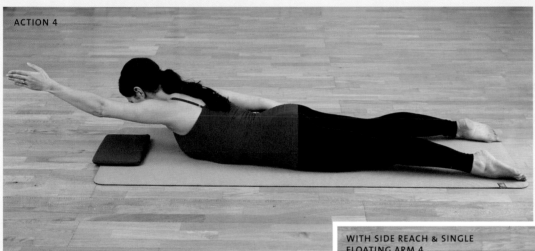

ACTION 4

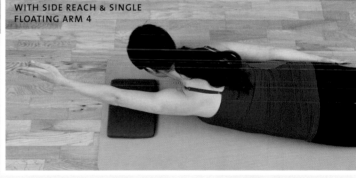

WITH SIDE REACH & SINGLE FLOATING ARM 4

DART WITH SIDE REACH AND SINGLE FLOATING ARM (LEVEL 4)

Adding a floating arm increases the load and thus the toning power of this exercise, which is a combination of Dart with Two Floating Arms and Dart with Side Reach. There's a lot going on, so try to stay in control of each component part.

STARTING POSITION

As for Dart (page 180) but with feet hip-width or, if more comfortable, shoulder-width apart.

ACTION

Follow Action Points 1 and 2 for Dart with Side Reach (opposite), then:

3 Breathe in and float your left arm up, turning the palm to face inward.

4 Breathe out as you sequentially side-bend to the right. Keep your pelvis central.

5 Breathe in and return to centre.

6 Breathe out and press your arm back down by your side.

7 Repeat 3 times to each side.

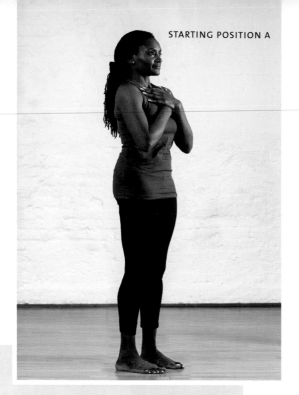

STARTING POSITION A

STANDING BACK BEND (LEVEL 4)

This is a wonderful exercise to finish your workouts. You could even do it during the day at the office to counter the effects of being hunched over a desk.

STARTING POSITION
Stand tall in Parallel (page 58). Either relax your hands by your sides, cross them over your chest or lightly clasp them behind your head (to support your neck). If clasping behind your head, keep your elbows in your peripheral vision.

ACTION

1 Breathe in and, initiating with your head, begin to gently bend backward sequentially, arching the spine evenly vertebra by vertebra. Aim for an even curve along the whole spine.

2 Breathe out and begin to restack your spine sequentially from bottom to top, lengthening as you do so.

3 Repeal up to 10 times.

STARTING POSITION A

STARTING POSITION B

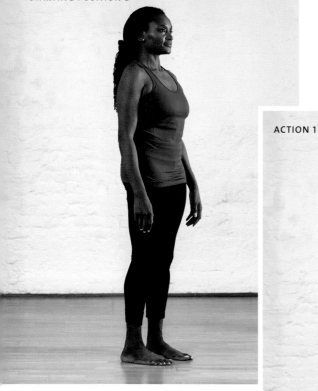

ACTION 1

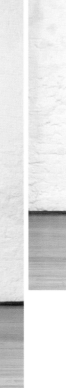

ACTION 1

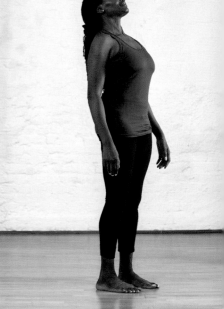

ACTION 1

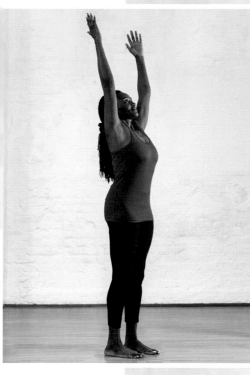

STANDING BACK BEND WITH ARM CIRCLES (LEVEL 4)

Once you are confident with your Standing Back Bends you can add Arm Circles. They feel sensational.

Circle your arms as you extend backwards, opening your chest. Time your circle so your arms are back alongside your body as you return to upright.

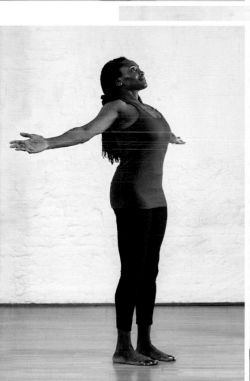

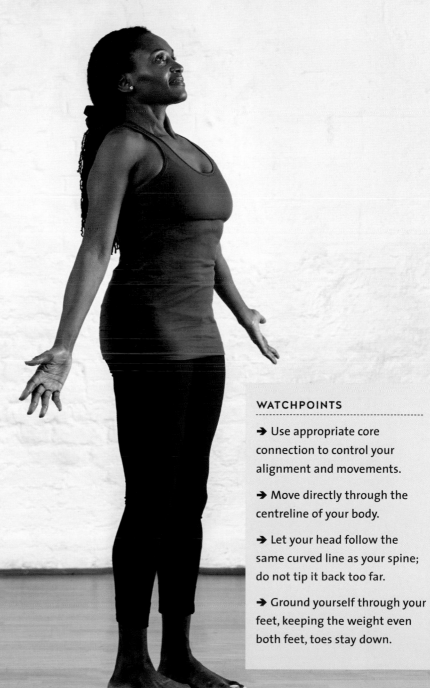

WATCHPOINTS

➜ Use appropriate core connection to control your alignment and movements.

➜ Move directly through the centreline of your body.

➜ Let your head follow the same curved line as your spine; do not tip it back too far.

➜ Ground yourself through your feet, keeping the weight even both feet, toes stay down.

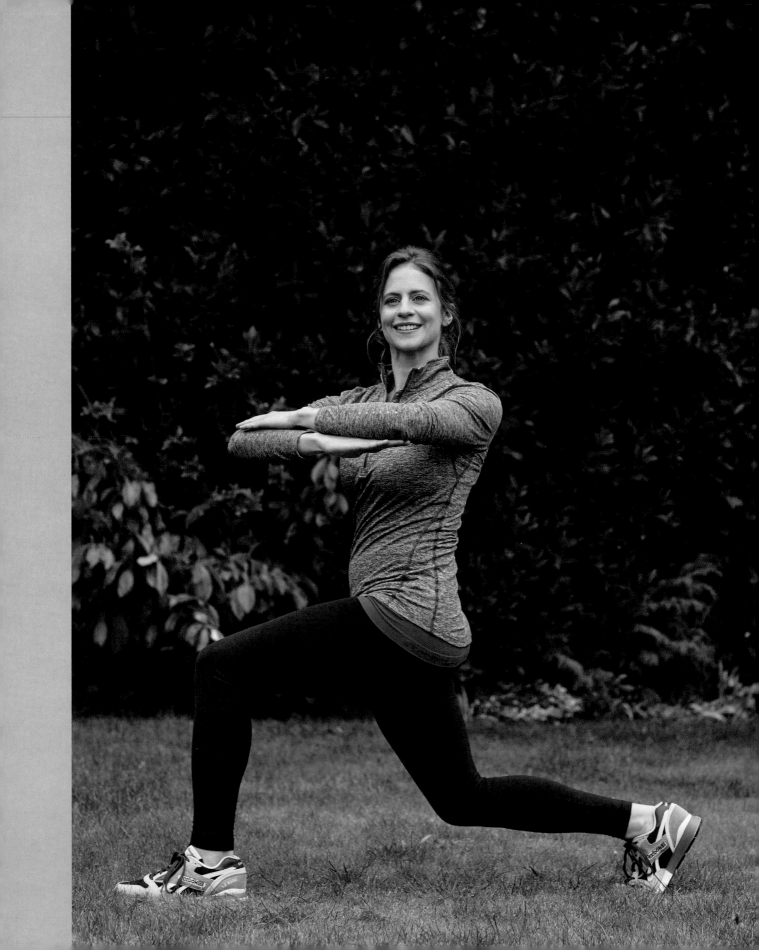

ADDING Cardio TO YOUR SHAPE UP Programme

HOW MUCH CARDIOVASCULAR EXERCISE?

Although Pilates is a fabulous body-conditioning method, it does not provide a cardiovascular workout. The notable exceptions are the Hundred (page 124) and some of the Dynamic Lunges (page 170) and Squats (page 168) we've created for you, but we would not recommend doing those continuously for 30 minutes.

For heart health, it's essential to add some cardiovascular activities to your weekly routine. The ideal combination would be 150 minutes (2½ hours) of Pilates practice a week with 150 minutes (2½ hours) of aerobic activities. Five hours of exercise every week! That seems a lot, but if you enjoy Pilates, pick fun aerobic activities and add incidental exercise into your daily activities (see page 190), it's doable!

What is a cardiovascular, or aerobic, activity? One that involves moving your whole body, especially if it engages the large muscles like those in the legs. During cardiovascular exercise, oxygen is needed to power the muscles. As you become aerobically fit, your body becomes more efficient at transporting oxygen. Cardiovascular activities also help to burn more calories, which is why Pilates and cardiovascular activity together form the perfect shape-up and weight-loss partnership.

The World Health Organization suggests that every week adults aged 18–64 should do at least 150 minutes of moderate aerobic activity, such as cycling or brisk walking, or 75 minutes of vigorous aerobic activity, like running or a game of singles tennis. Alternatively, you can mix moderate and vigorous aerobic activity – for example, two vigorous 30-minute runs plus 30 minutes of brisk walking equates to 150 minutes of moderate aerobic activity.

> ### BENEFITS OF CARDIOVASCULAR ACTIVITY
>
> - Strengthens the heart, lungs and circulatory system.
> - Reduces risk of heart disease.
> - Lowers blood pressure.
> - Improves blood cholesterol and triglyceride levels.
> - Releases endorphins (feel-good hormones), which in turn helps reduce stress levels and may help depression.
> - Improves muscle strength.
> - Aids weight-management.

How do you judge your level of activity? Moderate activities are those that cause your heart to beat faster and make you feel warmer. You should still be able to talk while exercising, but singing will be tricky. Vigorous activity makes you breathe hard and fast. If you're working at this level, you won't be able to say more than a few words without pausing for breath. In general, 75 minutes of vigorous activity can give similar health benefits to 150 minutes of moderate activity.

You need to decide what works best for you. Probably the optimum way to hit the recommended 150 minutes of weekly physical activity is to do 30 minutes on five days every week. If you plan at least three cardio sessions (moderate or vigorous) to your diary, it's then easy to hit the target by adding as many incidental cardiovascular activities as possible into your day. To stay motivated, choose cardiovascular activities you enjoy, which makes it easier to stick to a routine, and buddy up with a friend.

MODERATE-INTENSITY ACTIVITIES

- Brisk walking
- Water aerobics
- Riding a bike on level ground or with few hills
- Doubles tennis
- Pushing a lawn mower
- Hiking
- Skateboarding
- Rollerblading
- Volleyball
- Basketball

VIGOROUS-INTENSITY ACTIVITIES

- Jogging or running
- Swimming fast
- Riding a bike fast or on hills
- Singles tennis
- Squash
- Football
- Rugby
- Skipping
- Hockey
- Aerobics classes
- Gymnastics
- Martial arts

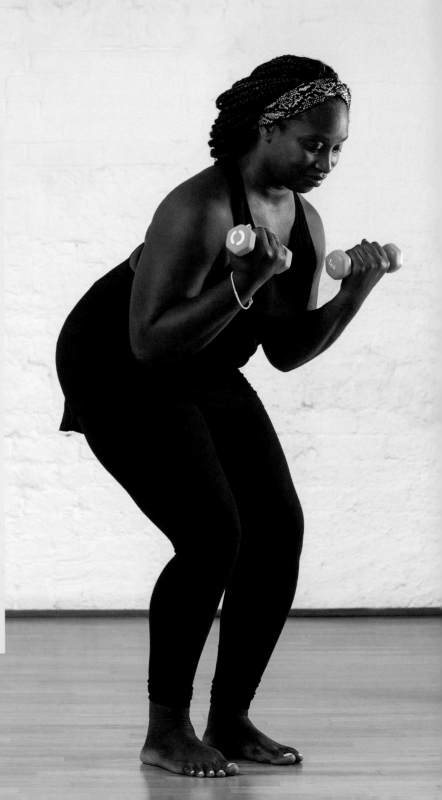

Working at the right intensity

It's important when doing cardiovascular exercise to track your heart rate. Start by working out your resting heart rate: the number of times your heart beats per minute when you are at rest (see box below). A good time to check is in the morning after a good night's sleep, and before drinking tea or coffee.

For most of us, between 60 and 100 beats per minute (bpm) is normal, but the rate can be affected by stress, anxiety, hormones, medication and how physically active you are. You may also find your training zone varies from day to day. If you are fit, your heart rate will be lower because your heart muscle is in better condition and doesn't have to work as hard to maintain a steady beat.

MAXIMUM TARGET HEART RATE

AGE	TARGET HEART RATE ZONE 50–85%	AVERAGE MAXIMUM HEART RATE 100%
20 years	100–170 beats per minute (bpm)	200 bpm
30 years	95–162 bpm	190 bpm
35 years	93–157 bpm	185 bpm
40 years	90–153 bpm	180 bpm
45 years	88–149 bpm	175 bpm
50 years	85–145 bpm	170 bpm
55 years	83–140 bpm	165 bpm
60 years	80–136 bpm	160 bpm
65 years	78–132 bpm	155 bpm
70 years	75–128 bpm	150 bpm

HOW TO WORK OUT YOUR HEART RATE

1 Press lightly over the artery on the inside of your wrist, on the thumb side, using the tips of your first two fingers (not your thumb).
2 Count your pulse for 30 seconds.
3 Multiply the count by 2 to find your beats per minute.

Once you know your resting heart rate, check it against the chart showing target heart-rate zones for different ages (left). Find the age category closest to yours and read across to see your target heart rate (the figures are averages, so use as a general guide).

During moderate intensity activities, aim for about 50–70 percent of your maximum heart rate; during vigorous physical activity, aim for 70–85 percent. Your maximum heart rate is about 220 minus your age. A fitness tracker will do the calculations for you, though take care as some trackers are more accurate than others.

If your heart rate is too high during exercising, you are working too hard. If it's too low, and the intensity feels light to moderate, you may want to push yourself a little harder, especially if you're trying to lose weight. If you have been inactive for a while, aim for the lower range of your target zone (50 percent), building up gradually. In time you'll be able to exercise comfortably at up to 85 percent of your maximum heart rate.

Getting more active – how incidental exercise makes hitting your targets easier

One of the most effective things you can do for heart health is to increase your overall levels of incidental activity. Long periods of sitting in particular are detrimental to health, and need breaking up with regular periods of activity.

You can also step your way to health and fitness. Aim for 4,000 steps a day (spread throughout the day) for general health, 7,000 steps to improve your fitness and 10,000 to lose weight. It's easy to log them on a phone app or fitness tracker. You'll need to do some research to see which brand is more accurate at counting steps.

Your pace needs to be fast enough to raise your heart rate for walking to count as a cardiovascular activity. At a slower pace, even taking 10,000 steps a day, you may fall short of the required amount of cardiovascular activity you need to maintain heart health.

EXERCISE SNACKING

There is interesting research into the benefits of breaking up exercise into short sessions.

A 2018 University of Bath, UK study suggested that just five minutes of exercise at home twice a day can lead to marked improvements in muscle mass and strength in older adults – in just four weeks they were able to rebuild the amount of muscle people of this age lose over 1–2 years. Participants did each exercise for one minute, completing as many repetitions as they could, then rested for one minute before doing the next exercise. After four weeks of this exercise "snacking", their number repetitions went up by 30 percent, while leg strength and power and thigh muscle size all

increased. The results are so incredible for such a short period that we have added short workouts in our Shape Up programme and extra repetitions to the exercises.

We have also included weights work – a 2018 study at Iowa State University in the USA revealed that lifting weights for less than an hour once a week may reduce the risk of heart attack or stroke by 40–70 percent. Spending longer than an hour weightlifting did not add any extra benefits.

WAYS TO ADD INCIDENTAL ACTIVITY TO YOUR DAY

- Walk to work rather than taking the train or bus, or get off a stop early and walk the rest of the way.
- Avoid the nearest parking spot; park far away from the station, shops or office.
- Walk to the farthest bus stop or station.
- Take the stairs not the lift.
- Walk, don't stand, on escalators or moving walkways at airports.
- During lunch breaks, walk around the block a few times before eating.
- Take short breaks at work by running your own errands.
- Walk as you talk on the phone.
- Don't send an email, go talk to your colleague.
- Play active, rather than sedentary, video games.

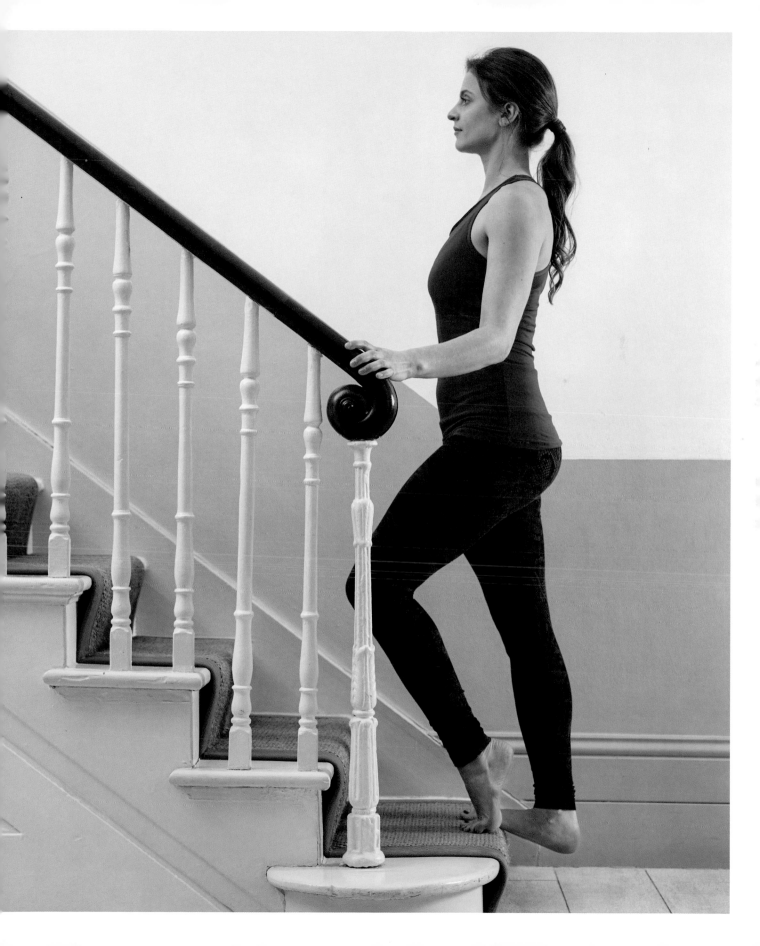

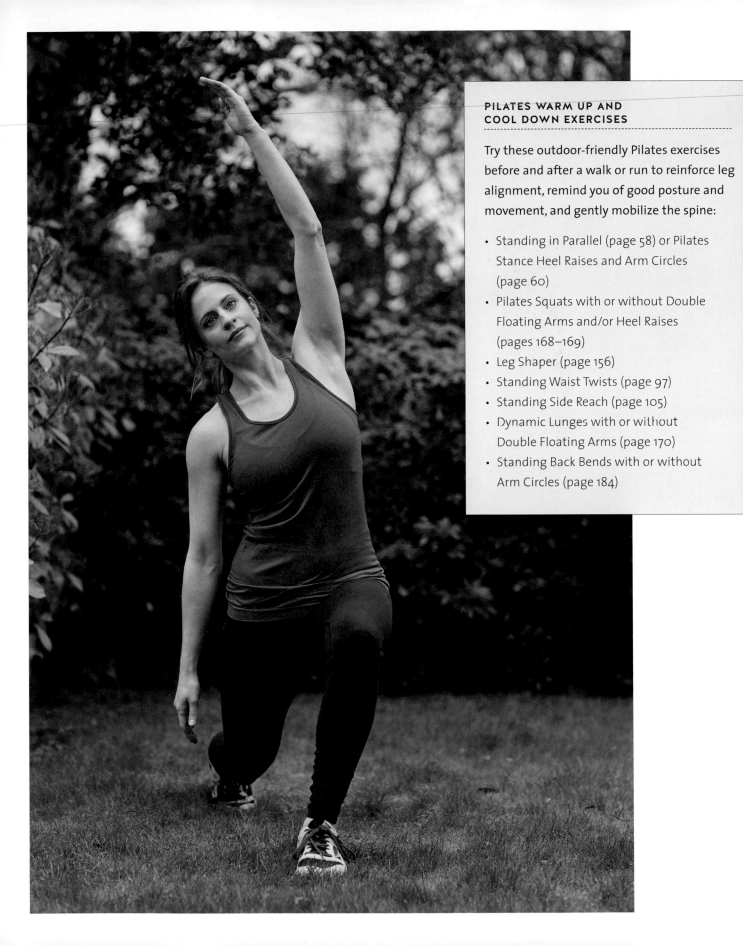

PILATES WARM UP AND COOL DOWN EXERCISES

Try these outdoor-friendly Pilates exercises before and after a walk or run to reinforce leg alignment, remind you of good posture and movement, and gently mobilize the spine:

- Standing in Parallel (page 58) or Pilates Stance Heel Raises and Arm Circles (page 60)
- Pilates Squats with or without Double Floating Arms and/or Heel Raises (pages 168–169)
- Leg Shaper (page 156)
- Standing Waist Twists (page 97)
- Standing Side Reach (page 105)
- Dynamic Lunges with or without Double Floating Arms (page 170)
- Standing Back Bends with or without Arm Circles (page 184)

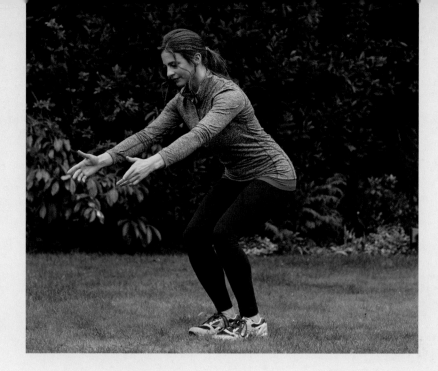

SAFE CARDIO EXERCISING

- Choose an activity or class to suit your level of fitness, physical limitations and needs.

- Whatever the form of exercise, stay mindful of your movements. Walk, jog and run tall.

- Do not attempt to stay connected to your core throughout an aerobic workout – it's not possible and will limit the freedom of your movements. However, you may remind yourself that your abdomen is not supposed to bulge.

- Check the qualifications of instructors and personal trainers.

- Dress appropriately for the weather, and wear a good supportive bra.

- Choose correct footwear, especially for running, to prevent shin splints and ankle injuries.

- Run with a friend if possible, and make sure someone knows your route and what time you are expected home.

- Stay alert to your surroundings. If you listen to music, keep the volume very low or use just one ear piece.

- Wear reflective clothing and face oncoming traffic when jogging on a road.

- Alternate walking on different sides of a road so the same leg isn't consistently on the downhill slope. When the downhill leg bends slightly inward, the iliotibial band (a ligament running along the outside of the thigh) stretches, which can cause irritation and pain.

- Watch the impact on your joints from surfaces. Concrete is less forgiving than asphalt, and cinder tracks or dirt trails softer and gentler on your joints.

- In the countryside, watch for uneven terrain, rocks, roots or hidden holes. You may need hiking shoes rather than trainers.

- Wear a protective helmet for cycling and check your lights are in order.

- Take plenty of water.

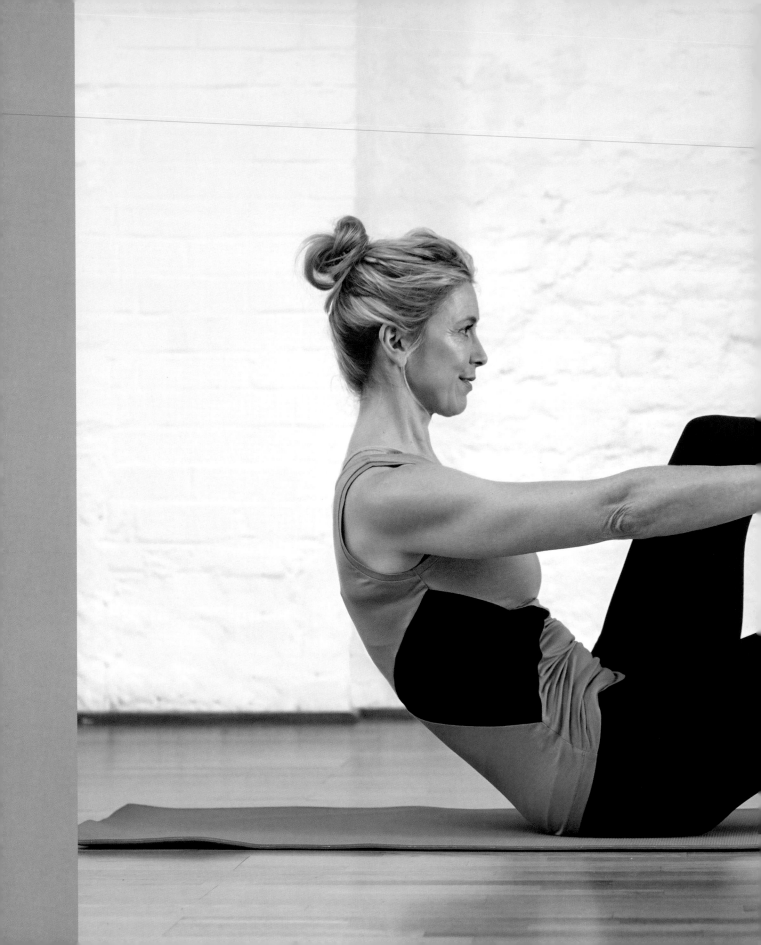

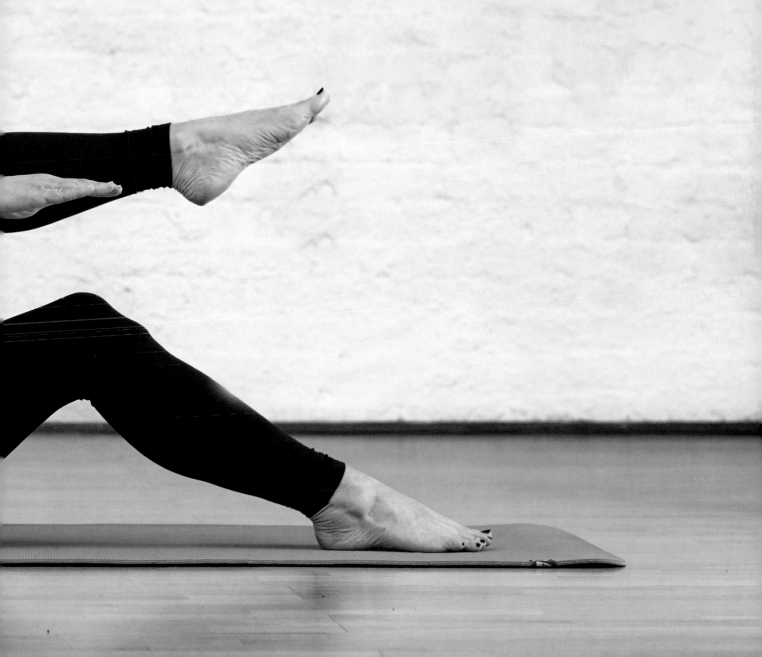

THE SHAPE UP
Workouts

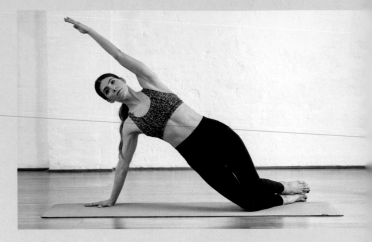

Here we go... this is what you've been waiting for, the fun bit where you get to enjoy the flow and challenge of a Pilates session in your own home. You will find workouts of varying lengths and levels of difficulty, and we've done all the calculations for you, so you don't have to waste time worrying what to do next.

You must decide how much time you can spare for Pilates, but your goal for maximum shape up is for your workouts to add up to about 150 minutes (2½ hours) a week. If you decide to take longer than 12 weeks to shape up, you could drop the workout time to 120 minutes or even 90 minutes a week. I wouldn't go lower than this or your body may not absorb all the movement skills you need and you may not tone up enough to change your metabolic rate and make a significant difference to your shape. You'll feel better, but we want you to look stunning.

We've labelled the workouts Shorter (10–15 minutes), Medium (25–30 minutes) and Longer (45–50 minutes). If you have only 10 minutes, just do a few repetitions of each exercise, adding more if you have more time. It's important to work precisely and mindfully, remembering your ABCs (see page 46).

All the workouts are balanced in terms of spinal movements, including flexion, rotation, side flexion and extension exercises – even in the short workouts. Longer workouts are better balanced in terms of upper and lower body toning.

We have saved the Arm Weights sequences for longer workouts. You could add them to the shorter workouts, but warm up the shoulders first with Arm Circles (page 84), Ribcage Closure (page 79) or Shoulder Drops (page 78). You can also add any of the Shape Up More and Shape Up Even More exercises for abdominals, waist, arms and buttocks to your workouts if these areas need more work.

We begin with workouts taken solely from the New Fundamentals – perfect if you are new to Pilates or want a simple workout. Sometimes my body craves this simplicity in the same way it may crave a simple omelette over a sophisticated dish.

When you feel confident with your strength, flexibility and movement control you can progress to the Level 1–3 workouts (there are lots at this level). And when you are ready, start adding in Level 4, 5 and 6 exercises, doing the workouts in rotation. Remember you can still do workouts from lower levels of difficulty.

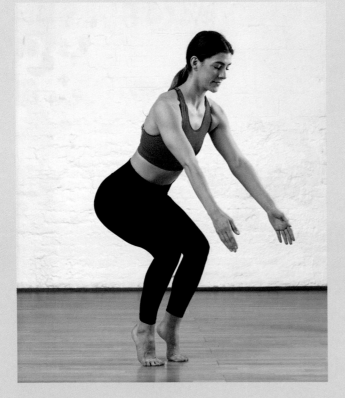

The New Fundamentals workouts level 1–2

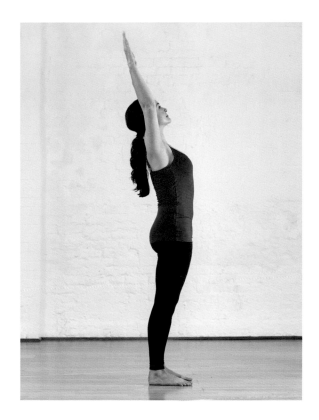

To get you started here are 10 balanced workouts made up exclusively of exercises from the New Fundamentals chapter. They are 25–30 minutes in length, the perfect length of time for your body to "absorb" the ABCs and complete the full number of repetitions to learn new skills. If you have more time, blend two workouts together.

There is quite a lot of repetition in these workouts. This is deliberate to really reinforce your understanding of the exercises. Relaxation Position, Chin Tucks and Neck Rolls feature in every workout to mobilize your neck gently before you attempt Curl Ups and abdominal work. Rest Position usually follows back extension work.

WORKOUT 1
- Relaxation Position (page 48): The Compass (page 50), Chin Tucks and Neck Rolls (page 52)
- Shoulder Drops (page 78)
- Single Knee Folds (page 69)
- Spine Curls (page 90)
- Hip Rolls (page 102)
- Curl Ups (page 92)
- Arm Openings (page 100)
- Oyster (page 87)
- Diamond Press (page 106)
- Table Top Level 1 (page 74)
- Rest Position with Deep Abdominal Breathing (page 108)
- High Kneeling Single Floating Arms (page 82)
- Standing Side Reach (page 104)
- Standing Heel Raises (page 60)
- Pilates Squat (page 168)

WORKOUT 2
- Standing Pilates Stance (page 60)
- Standing Double Floating Arms (page 83)
- Standing Waist Twist (page 97)
- Relaxation Position (page 48): The Compass (page 50), Chin Tucks and Neck Rolls (page 52)
- Deep Abdominal Breathing (page 63)
- Knee Openings (page 69)
- Spine Curls (page 90)
- Curl Ups (page 92)
- Hip Rolls (page 102)
- Oyster (page 87)
- Diamond Press (page 106)
- Cat (page 95)
- Rest Position (page 108)
- High Kneeling Lunge Position (page 56, Scarf Breathing, page 62, in this position, swapping legs after a few breaths)
- Standing Side Reach (page 104)
- Pilates Stance Heel Raises (page 60)

WORKOUT 3

- Seated Scarf Breathing (page 62)
- Seated Side Reach (page 104)
- Relaxation Position (page 48): The Compass (page 50), Chin Tucks and Neck Rolls (page 52)
- Double Shoulder Drops (page 78)
- Leg Slides (page 68)
- Spine Curls (page 90)
- Curl Ups (page 92)
- Butterflies (page 101)
- Diamond Press (page 106)
- Star Prep (page 85)
- Cat (page 95)
- Rest Position (page 108)
- Standing Double Floating Arms (page 83)
- Standing Waist Twist (page 97)
- Pilates Squat (page 168)

WORKOUT 4

- Relaxation Position (page 48): The Compass (page 50), Chin Tucks and Neck Rolls (page 52)
- The Hundred Level 1 Breathing (page 63)
- Knee Fold and Extend (page 71)
- Arm Circles (page 84)
- Knee Rolls (page 73)
- Spine Curls (page 90)
- Curl Ups (page 92)
- Hip Rolls (page 102)
- Oyster with Band (page 88)
- Diamond Press (page 106)
- Table Top Level 1 (page 74)
- Rest Position (page 108)
- High Kneeling Waist Twist (page 97)
- Standing Side Reach (page 104)
- Pilates Squat (page 168)

WORKOUT 5

- Standing Pilates Stance (page 60)
- Standing Waist Twist (page 97)
- Standing Side Reach (page 104)
- Relaxation Position (page 48): Chin Tucks and Neck Rolls (page 52)
- Deep Abdominal Breathing (page 63)
- Arm Circles (page 84)
- Knee Fold and Extend (page 71)
- Spine Curls (page 90)
- Curl Ups with Leg Slide (page 93)
- Hip Rolls (page 102)
- Arm Openings (page 100)
- Diamond Press (page 106)
- Cat (page 95)
- Rest Position (page 108)
- Seated C-Curve (page 94)
- Ribcage Closure against a Wall (page 80)
- Roll Downs against a Wall (page 110)

WORKOUT 6

- Relaxation Position (page 48): The Compass (page 50), Chin Tucks and Neck Rolls (page 52)
- The Hundred Level 1 Breathing (page 63)
- Knee Openings (page 69)
- Ribcage Closure (page 79)
- Spine Curls (page 90)
- Curl Ups (page 92)
- Arm Openings (page 100)
- Diamond Press (page 106)
- Table Top Level 1 (page 74)
- Rest Position (page 108)
- High Kneeling Side Reach (page 104)
- Standing Heel Raises (page 60)
- Pilates Squat (page 168)

WORKOUT 7

- Seated Long Frog (page 53): Scarf Breathing (page 62)
- Seated Side Reach (page 104)
- Relaxation Position (page 48): Chin Tucks, Neck Rolls (page 52), Deep Abdominal Breathing (page 63)
- Double Shoulder Drops (page 78)
- Curl Ups with Leg Slide (page 93)
- Hip Rolls (page 102)
- Butterflies (page 101)
- Star Prep (page 85)
- Diamond Press (page 106)
- Cat (page 95)
- Rest Position (page 108)
- High Kneeling Double Floating Arms (page 83)
- Standing Waist Twist (page 97)
- Standing Heel Raises (page 60)
- Roll Downs against a Wall (page 110)

WORKOUT 8

- Standing Pilates Stance (page 60)
- Heel Raises (page 60)
- Double Floating Arms (page 83)
- Standing Waist Twist (page 97)
- Relaxation Position (page 48): Chin Tucks and Neck Rolls (page 52)
- Spine Curls (page 90)
- Ribcage Closure (page 79)
- Curl Ups (page 92)
- Arm Openings (page 100)
- Diamond Press (page 106)
- Table Top Level 1 or 2 (page 74)
- Rest Position (page 108)
- High Kneeling Scarf Breathing (page 62)
- Standing Side Reach (page 104)
- Pilates Squat (page 168)

WORKOUT 9

- Relaxation Position (page 48): Chin Tucks and Neck Rolls (page 52)
- The Hundred Level 1 Breathing (page 63)
- Arm Circles (page 84)
- Knee Fold and Extend (page 71)
- Spine Curls (page 90)
- Curl Ups with Leg Slide (page 93)
- Oyster with Band (page 88)
- Butterflies (page 101)
- Diamond Press (page 106)
- Cat (page 95)
- Rest Position (page 108)
- High Kneeling Side Reach (page 94)
- Standing Waist Twist (page 97)
- Pilates Squat (page 168)
- Roll Downs against a Wall (page 110)

WORKOUT 10

- Standing Heel Raises (page 60)
- Standing Side Reach (page 104)
- High Kneeling Waist Twist (page 97)
- Relaxation Position (page 48): Chin Tucks and Neck Rolls (page 52)
- Deep Abdominal Breathing (page 63)
- Shoulder Drops (page 78)
- Arm Circles (page 84)
- Spine Curls (page 90)
- Curl Ups (page 92)
- Hip Rolls (page 102)
- Butterflies (page 101)
- Diamond Press (page 106)
- Table Top Level 2 (page 75)
- Rest Position (page 108)
- Seated C-Curve (page 94)
- Ribcage Closure against a Wall with Wall Slide (page 81)
- Pilates Squat (page 168)

Workouts level 1–3

Now you have mastered the New Fundamentals you can move on to add more challenging (and therefore more toning) exercises. Here you will find 10 short balanced workouts for Levels 1–3. Do them in rotation, adding a longer workout when you have more time.

If an exercise has several levels of difficulty, choose the right level for you. When in doubt, select the simplest version of exercises until you are ready for the complex combinations.

Shorter workouts level 1–3
(10–15 MINUTES)

There are 12–13 exercises in each of these workouts. If you only have 10 minutes to spare, do a few repetitions of each exercise.

WORKOUT 1
· Relaxation Position (page 48):
  Chin Tucks and Neck Rolls (page 52)
· Deep Abdominal Breathing (page 63)
· Arm Circles (page 84)
· Knee Rolls (page 73, arms up in Shoulder Drop position)
· Basic Bridge (page 158)
· Oblique Curl Ups (page 116)
· Arm Openings with Weights (page 101)
· Dart (page 180)
· Cat (page 95)
· Rest Position (page 108)
· Standing Side Reach (page 104)
· Dynamic Backward Lunge (page 170)
· Roll Downs (page 110)

WORKOUT 2
· Standing Pilates Stance with Heel Raises (page 60)
· Standing Side Reach (page 104)
· Relaxation Position (page 48):
  Chin Tucks and Neck Rolls (page 52)
· Ribcage Closure (page 79)
· The Hundred Breathing Pattern (page 63)
· Spine Curls (page 90)
· Curl Ups with Knee Openings (page 93)
· Side Kick Series: Small Circles (page 141)
· Cobra Prep (page 174)
· Table Top Level 2 (page 75)
· Rest Position (page 108)
· High Kneeling Lunge Waist Twist (page 98)
· Pilates Squat (page 168)

WORKOUT 3
· Ribcage Closure against a Wall with Wall Slide (page 81)
· High Kneeling Side Reach (page 104)
· Relaxation Position (page 48):
  Chin Tucks and Neck Rolls (page 52)
· Shoulder Drops (page 78)
· Basic Bridge (page 158)
· Oblique Curl Ups with Knee Fold (page 117)
· Arm Openings with Weights (page 101)
· Dart (page 180)
· One-armed Cat (page 96)
· Rest Position with Deep Abdominal Breathing (page 108)
· Pelvic Roll Backs (page 130)
· Wall Push Ups (page 146)
· Pilates Squats with Heel Raise (page 169)

WORKOUT 4

- Relaxation Position (page 48): Chin Tucks and Neck Rolls (page 52)
- Double Shoulder Drops (page 78)
- Spine Curls with Knee Opening (page 91)
- Oblique Curl Ups with Reach (page 117)
- Hip Rolls (page 102, if ready, with Leg Extension, page 103)
- Side-lying Knee Cross Overs (page 89)
- Cobra Prep (page 174)
- Table Top with Arm Salute (page 76)
- Rest Position (page 108)
- High Kneeling Lunge Side Reach (page 105)
- High Kneeling Scarf Breathing (page 62)
- Pilates Squats with Bicep Curls (page 169)
- Roll Downs (page 110)

WORKOUT 5

- Standing Pilates Stance with Double Floating Arms (page 83)
- Standing Side Reach (page 104)
- Relaxation Position (page 48): Chin Tucks and Neck Rolls (page 52)
- The Hundred Breathing Pattern (page 63)
- Basic Bridge (page 158)
- Oblique Curl Ups with Knee Fold (page 117)
- Double Leg Stretch Prep (page 122)
- Side Kick Series: Small Circles (page 141)
- Dart (page 180)
- Cat (page 95)
- Rest Position (page 108)
- High Kneeling Lunge Waist Twist (page 98)
- Roll Downs with Weights (page 112)

WORKOUT 6

- Relaxation Position (page 48): Chin Tucks and Neck Rolls (page 52)
- Knee Rolls with Ribcage Closure (page 73)
- Spine Curls with Arm Circles (page 91)
- Curl Ups with Single Knee Fold (page 93)
- The Hundred – your level (page 124)
- Hip Rolls (page 102, if ready, adding Leg Extension, page 103)
- Torpedo Prep (page 142)
- Dart with Side Reach (page 182)
- Box Push Ups (page 150)
- Rest Position (page 108)
- Pelvic Roll Backs (page 130)
- Dynamic Backward, or Forward Lunges with Biceps Curls (page 173)
- Pilates Squat (page 168)

WORKOUT 7

- Pilates Squats with Heel Raises (page 169)
- Standing Arm Circles (page 84)
- Standing Waist Twist (page 97)
- Relaxation Position (page 48): Chin Tucks and Neck Rolls (page 52)
- Spine Curls with Arm Circles (page 91)
- Single Leg Stretch Toe Taps (page 120)
- Oblique Curl Ups with Reach (page 117)
- Side Twist Prep (page 138)
- Dart with Side Reach (page 182)
- One-armed Cat (page 96)
- Rest Position with Deep Abdominal Breathing (page 108)
- Back Bridge (page 162)
- Roll Downs with Weights (page 112)

WORKOUT 8

- Seated Long Frog (page 53): Waist Twists (page 97)
- Seated Scarf Breathing (page 62)
- Relaxation Position (page 48): Chin Tucks and Neck Rolls (page 52)
- Shoulder Drops (page 78)
- Bridge with Band (page 159)
- Curl Ups with Knee Opening (page 93)
- The Hundred – your level (page 124)
- Torpedo Prep (page 142)
- Dart with Side Reach (page 182)
- Box Push Ups (page 150)
- Rest Position (page 108)
- Pelvic Roll Backs with Leg Slide (page 131)
- Dynamic Lunges with Bicep Curls (page 173)
- Roll Downs (page 110)

WORKOUT 9

- Relaxation Position (page 48): Chin Tucks and Neck Rolls (page 52)
- Knee Rolls with Ribcage Closure (page 73)
- Spine Curls with Knee Openings (page 91)
- The Hundred Breathing Pattern (page 63)
- Curl Ups with Single Knee Fold (page 93)
- Oblique Curl Ups with Reach (page 117)
- Butterflies (page 101)
- Diamond Press Salute (page 107)
- Four-point Kneeling Flies (page 144)
- Rest Position (page 108)
- High Kneeling Lunge Side Reach (page 105)
- Dynamic with Double Floating Arms (page 172)
- Roll Downs with Weights (page 112)

WORKOUT 10

- Ribcage Closure with Wall Slide (page 81)
- Standing Waist Twist (page 97)
- Relaxation Position (page 48): Chin Tucks and Neck Rolls (page 52)
- Bridge with Band (page 159)
- Curl Ups with Knee Opening (page 93)
- Double Leg Stretch Prep (page 122)
- Side Twist Prep (page 138)
- Lizard (page 178)
- Cat (page 95)
- Rest Position with Deep Abdominal Breathing (page 108)
- Pelvic Roll Backs with Leg Slide (page 131)
- Standing Side Reach (page 104)
- Pilates Squats with Band (page 169)

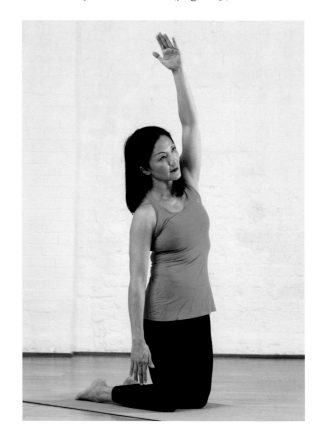

Medium workouts level 1–3
(25–30 MINUTES)

Here are seven slightly longer workouts with 17–18 exercises to try. You should have time for a few more repetitions than with the shorter workouts. Do the workouts in rotation, as before, choosing the right level of difficulty for you.

With a bit more time available you can add some Deep Abdominal Breathing (page 63) to your workouts, if you wish.

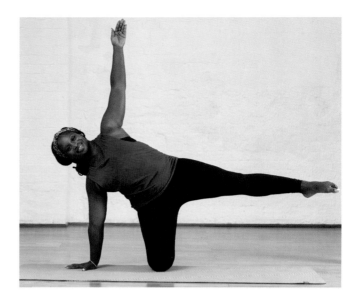

WORKOUT 1
- Relaxation Position (page 48): Chin Tucks and Neck Rolls (page 52)
- Shoulder Drops (page 78)
- Spine Curls with Ribcage Closure (page 91)
- Hip Rolls (page 102)
- Curl Ups with Leg Slide (page 93)
- Oblique Curl Ups with Reach (page 117)
- The Hundred – your level (page 124)
- Arm Openings with Weights (page 101)
- Side-lying Knee Cross Overs (page 89)
- Cobra Prep (page 174)
- Table Top Level 2 (page 75)
- Rest Position (page 108)
- Pelvic Roll Backs (page 130)
- High Kneeling Lunge Side Reach (page 105)
- Standing Arm Weights Sequence: Biceps Press, Chest Expansion (page 153)
- Pilates Squats with Heel Raise (page 169)

WORKOUT 2
- Standing Pilates Stance with Arm Circles (page 84)
- Pilates Squats with Band around Thighs (page 169)
- Standing Side Reach (page 104)
- High Kneeling Lunge Waist Twist (page 98)
- Relaxation Position (page 48): Chin Tucks and Neck Rolls (page 52)
- Knee Rolls with Ribcage Closure (page 73)
- Bridge with Band (page 159)
- Hip Rolls with Leg Extension (page 103)
- Curl Ups with Single Knee Folds (page 93)
- Double Leg Stretch Prep (page 122)
- Butterflies (page 101)
- Torpedo Prep (page 142)
- Dart (page 180)
- Star Prep (page 85)
- Cat (page 95)
- Rest Position with Deep Abdominal Breathing (page 108)
- Wall Push Ups (page 146)
- Dynamic Forward Lunges with Bicep Curls (page 173)
- Roll Downs with Weights (page 112)

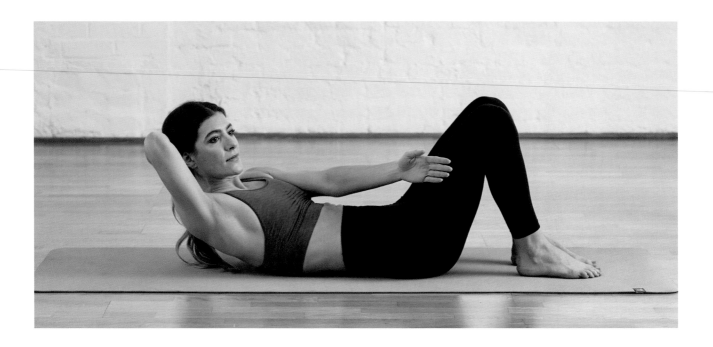

WORKOUT 3

WORKOUT 4

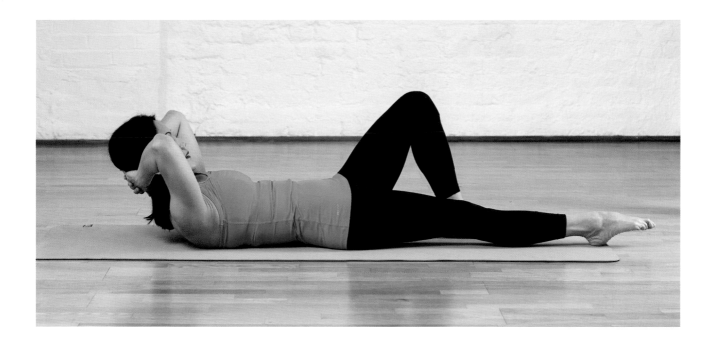

WORKOUT 5

WORKOUT 6

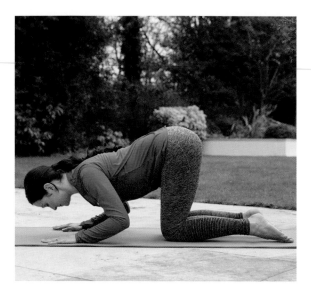

WORKOUT 7

- Pilates Stance with Heel Raises (page 60)
- Standing Arm Circles (page 84)
- Standing Waist Twist (page 97)
- One Arm Wall Push Ups (page 147)
- Relaxation Position (page 48):
  Chin Tucks and Neck Rolls (page 52)
- Knee Rolls with Ribcage Closure (page 73)
- Bridge with Band (page 159)
- Curl Ups with Leg Slide (page 93)
- Oblique Curl Ups with Knee Fold (page 117)
- The Hundred – your level (page 124)
- Torpedo (page 143)
- Dart (page 180)
- Star Prep (page 85)
- Cat (page 95)
- Table Top Level 2 (page 75)
- Rest Position (page 108)
- Pelvic Roll Backs (page 130)
- High Kneeling Lunge Side Reach (page 105)
- Pilates Squats with Bicep Curls (page 169)
- Dynamic Lunges with Double Floating Arms (page 172)
- Roll Downs (page 110)

Longer workouts level 1–3
(45–50 MINUTES)

There are around 22 exercises in each of these workouts. Do the full number of suggested repetitions if you can for maximum results. Add any extra abdominal, buttocks or arm exercises to the middle section of the workout once your joints are warmed up properly.

As before, you can add some Deep Abdominal Breathing (page 63) whenever you feel the need for release.

WORKOUT 1

- Relaxation Position (page 48):
  Chin Tucks and Neck Rolls (page 52)
- Shoulder Drops (page 78)
- Knee Rolls with Ribcage Closure (page 73)
- Spine Curls (page 90)
- Curl Ups with Leg Slide (page 93)
- Oblique Curl Ups with Reach (page 117)
- Single Leg Stretch Toe Taps (page 120)
- Hip Rolls (page 102)
- Oyster with Band (page 88)
- Torpedo Prep (page 142)
- Arm Openings with Weights (page 101)
- Lizard (page 178)
- Diamond Press with Leg Lift (page 107)
- One-armed Cat (page 96)
- Four-point Kneeling Flies (page 144)
- Rest Position with Deep Abdominal Breathing (page 108)
- Seated Long Frog (page 53): Waist Twist (page 96)
- Pelvic Roll Backs with Single Leg Slide (page 131)
- Back Bridge (page 162)
- High Kneeling Lunge Side Reach (page 105)
- Dynamic Lunge with Double Floating Arms (page 172)
- Leg Shaper (page 156)
- Roll Downs with Weights (page 112)

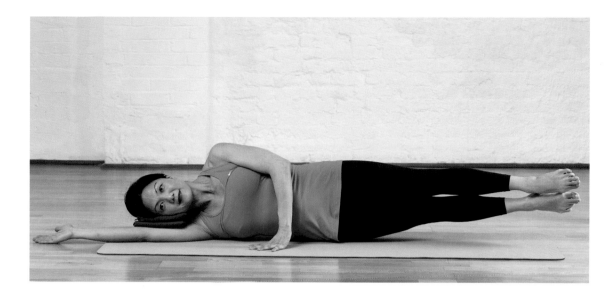

WORKOUT 2

- Pilates Stance with Heel Raises (page 60)
- Standing Arm Circles (page 84)
- Standing Side Reach (page 104)
- Relaxation Position (page 48): Chin Tucks and Neck Rolls (page 52)
- The Hundred Breathing Pattern (page 63)
- Ribcage Closure (page 79)
- Knee Fold and Extended Arms (page 72)
- Bridge with Band (page 159)
- Hip Rolls (page 102)
- Curl Ups with Knee Opening (page 93)
- Oblique Curl Ups (page 117)
- Double Leg Stretch Prep (page 122)
- Butterflies (page 101)
- Side Kick Series: Small Circles (page 141)
- Side Twist Prep (page 138)
- Cobra Prep (page 174)
- Dart with One Floating Arm (page 181)
- Cat (page 95)
- Box Push Ups (page 150)
- Rest Position (page 108)
- Back Bridge (page 162)
- High Kneeling Lunge Waist Twist (page 98)
- Dynamic Lunges with Bicep Curls (page 173)
- Roll Downs with Weights (page 112)

WORKOUT 3

- Ribcage Closure with Wall Slide (page 81)
- High Kneeling Side Reach (page 104)
- Relaxation Position (page 48): Chin Tucks and Neck Rolls (page 52)
- Shoulder Drops (page 78)
- Spine Curls with Arm Circles (page 91)
- Curl Ups with Leg Slide (page 93)
- Oblique Curl Ups with Knee Fold (page 117)
- The Hundred – your level (page 124)
- Arm Openings with Weights (page 101)
- Side-lying Knee Cross Overs (page 89)
- Torpedo Prep (page 142)
- Diamond Press Salute (page 107)
- Dart with One Floating Arm (page 181)
- Table Top with Arm Salute (page 76)
- Cat (page 95)
- Rest Position (page 108)
- Arm Weights Sequence: Bicep Curls, Chest Presses, Backstroke Arms, Flies (page 151)
- Pelvic Roll Backs with Leg Slide (page 131)
- High Kneeling Lunge Waist Twist (page 98)
- Dynamic Lunges with Double Floating Arms (page 172)
- Pilates Squat (page 168)

WORKOUT 4

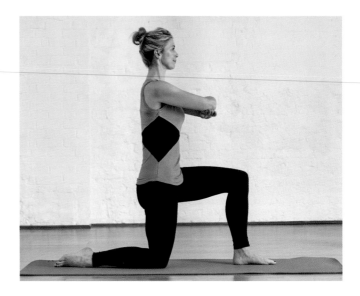

- Seated Long Frog (page 53): Waist Twist (page 96)
- Double Floating Arms (page 83)
- Seated Scarf Breathing (page 62)
- Relaxation Position (page 48): Chin Tucks and Neck Rolls (page 52)
- Shoulder Drops (page 78)
- Knee Rolls with Ribcage Closure (page 73)
- Bridge with Band (page 159)
- Spine Curls (page 90)
- Hip Rolls with Leg Extension (page 103)
- Curl Ups with Single Knee Folds (page 93)
- Oblique Curl Ups with Reach (page 117)
- Double Leg Stretch Prep (page 122)
- Butterflies (page 101)
- Side Twist Prep (page 138)
- Side Kick Series: Small Circles (page 141)
- Lizard (page 178)
- Dart with Side Reach (page 182)
- Star Prep Knee Lifts (page 85)
- Rest Position (page 108)
- Box Push Ups (page 150)
- Cat (page 95)
- C-Curve (page 94)
- Back Bridge (page 162)
- High Kneeling Lunge Side Reach (page 105)
- Dynamic Lunges with Bicep Curls (page 173)
- Pilates Squats with Band (page 169)
- Roll Downs with Weights (page 112)

WORKOUT 5

- Relaxation Position (page 48): Chin Tucks and Neck Rolls (page 52)
- Shoulder Drops (page 78)
- Arm Circles (page 84)
- Spine Curls with Knee Opening (page 91)
- Curl Ups with Leg Slides (page 93)
- Oblique Curl Ups (page 117)
- Single Leg Stretch Toe Taps (page 120)
- Hip Rolls (page 102)
- The Hundred Level 3 (page 126)
- Butterflies (page 101)
- Oyster with Band (page 88)
- Torpedo (page 143)
- Diamond Press Salute (page 107)
- Star Prep Knee Lifts (page 85)
- One-armed Cat (page 96)
- Table Top with Knee Bend (page 77)
- Rest Position with Deep Abdominal Breathing (page 108)
- Pelvic Roll Backs with Leg Slide (page 131)
- High Kneeling Lunge Side Reach (page 105)
- Dynamic Lunges (page 170)
- Standing Hand Weights Sequence: Biceps Press, Chest Expansion (page 153–155)
- Pilates Squats with Heel Raise (page 169)

Workouts level 1–5

Rather than giving you more workouts with exercises covering Levels 3–5, we suggest you add the more difficult exercises to the Level 1–3 workouts. We all progress at our own pace in movement skills, strength and flexibility so you must decide when you are ready for the more challenging levels. To help, here are the Level 4–5 exercises not yet included in your workouts. Add them when you feel ready.

LEVEL 4 EXERCISES

- Hip Rolls with Ribcage Closure (page 103)
- Table Top Arm Salute and Knee Bend (page 77)
- Table Top with Weights and Lifted Leg (page 145)
- Standing Single Floating Arms with Weights (page 83)
- Side-lying Knee Crosses Arms Overhead (page 88)
- Spine Curls with Knee Fold (page 91)
- Spine Curls with Knee Openings, Arms Up (page 91)
- Waist Twist in Static Standing Lunge (page 98)
- Static Standing Lunge Side Reach (page 105)
- Diamond Press Salute and Leg Lift (page 107)
- Roll Downs and Heel Raise (page 112)
- Oblique Curl Ups with Further Reach (page 117)
- Single Leg Stretch (page 121)
- Diamond Leg Lowers (page 128)
- Pelvic Roll Backs with Knee Fold (page 132)
- Pelvic Roll Backs with Bicep Curls (page 134)
- Pelvic Roll Backs with Rowing Prep and Variation (page 135)
- Dynamic Side Twist Prep (page 139)
- Side Kick Series: Small Circles (page 141, hands overhead)
- Torpedo Hamstring Curl (page 143)

- Torpedo Leg Lifts (page 143)
- One Arm Box Push Ups (page 150)
- Leg Pull Front Prep (page 148)
- Leg Shaper with Double Floating Arms (page 157)
- Bridge wand Knee Fold (page 159)
- Pretzel Bridge (page 160)
- Dynamic Lunges with Double Floating Arms and Weights (page 173)
- Full Cobra (page 176)
- Lizard with Legs (page 179)
- Dart with Two Floating Arms (page 181)
- Prone Beats (page 177)
- Standing Back Bend (page 184)
- Standing Back Bend with Arm Circles (page 185)
- The Hundred Level 4 (page 126)

LEVEL 5 EXERCISES

- Double Leg Stretch (page 123)
- Diamond Leg Lowers (page 129, hands behind head)
- Pelvic Roll Backs Double Leg Slide (page 132)
- Pelvic Roll Backs with Rotation (page 136)
- Criss Cross (page 118)
- The Hundred Level 5 (page 127)
- Bridge and Knee Fold and Extend (page 159)
- Back Bridge and Knee Fold and Extend (page 163)
- Pretzel Back Bridge (page 164)
- Leg Pull Back Prep (page 166)
- Dynamic Side Twist Prep 2 (page 140)
- Pretzel Bridge on Toes (page 161)
- Torpedo (page 143, hands off)
- Waist Twist in a Not So Static Standing Lunge (page 99)
- Dart with Simultaneous Double Floating Arms (page 181)

Workouts level 1–6

Here are workouts to really challenge you. There's a big difference between Level 4 and 6 so take it steady and work at the right level for you. When doing harder exercises it is even more important that your joints are gently mobilized at the start of a workout. Do not be tempted to skip these exercises!

Shorter workouts level 1–6
(10–15 MINUTES)

It's not easy to prepare for a Level 6 exercise in 10 minutes, so the shorter workouts do not include the higher levels of difficulty. But they still give you a challenging workout.

WORKOUT 1
- Relaxation Position (page 48): Chin Tucks and Neck Rolls (page 52)
- Knee Rolls with Ribcage Closure (page 73)
- Spine Curls with Knee Opening (page 91)
- Hip Rolls with Leg Extension (page 103)
- Curl Ups with Double Knee Fold (page 93)
- Oblique Curl Ups with Further Reach (page 117)
- The Hundred (page 124)
- Torpedo (page 143)
- Dart with Side Reach (page 182)
- One-armed Cat (page 96)
- Rest Position (page 108)
- High Kneeling Lunge Side Reach (page 105)
- Roll Downs with Weights (page 112)

WORKOUT 2
- Pilates Stance with Arm Circles and Heel Raise (page 60)
- High Kneeling Side Reach (page 104)
- Scarf Breathing (page 62)
- Relaxation Position (page 48): Chin Tucks and Neck Rolls (page 52)
- Basic Bridge (page 158)
- Oblique Curl Ups with Reach (page 117)
- Double Leg Stretch Prep (page 122)
- Diamond Leg Lowers (page 128)
- Butterflies (page 101)
- Lizard (page 178)
- Table Top with Flies (page 145)
- Rest Position (page 108)
- Pelvic Roll Backs with Knee Fold (page 132)
- Dynamic Lunges with Bicep Curls (page 173)

WORKOUT 3
- Ribcage Closure with Wall Slide and Heel Raise (page 81)
- Relaxation Position (page 48): Chin Tucks and Neck Rolls (page 52)
- Spine Curls with Arm Circles (page 91)
- Curl Ups with Double Knee Fold (page 93)
- The Hundred – your level (page 124)
- Arm Openings with Weights (page 101)
- Half Star (page 86)
- Cat (page 95)
- Rest Position (page 108)
- Back Bridge (page 162)
- High Kneeling Lunge Side Reach (page 105)
- Dynamic Lunges with Double Floating Arms (page 172)
- Roll Downs with Weights (page 112)

WORKOUT 4

- Seated Long Frog (page 53): Waist Twist (page 97)
- Relaxation Position (page 48): Chin Tucks and Neck Rolls (page 52)
- Hip Rolls with Ribcage Closure (page 103)
- Oblique Curl Ups with Reach (page 117)
- Single Leg Stretch Toe Taps (page 120)
- Side-lying Knee Cross Overs (page 89)
- Cobra Prep (page 174) or Full Cobra (page 176)
- Table Top with Arm Salute and Knee Bend (page 77)
- Rest Position with Deep Abdominal Breathing (page 108)
- Back Bridge (page 162)
- Pelvic Roll Backs (page 130)
- Static Standing Lunge Side Reach (page 105)
- Pilates Squats with Band (page 169)

WORKOUT 5

- Relaxation Position (page 48): Chin Tucks and Neck Rolls (page 52)
- Arm Circles (page 84)
- Spine Curls with Knee Openings (page 91)
- Curl Ups with Double Knee Fold (page 93)
- Double Leg Stretch Prep (page 122)
- The Hundred (page 124)
- Butterflies (page 101)
- Dart with Side Reach (page 182)
- High Kneeling Lunge Waist Twist (page 98)
- Pilates Squats with Band (page 169)
- Roll Downs with Weights and Heel Raises (page 112)

WORKOUT 6

- Pilates Stance with Heel Raise and Double Floating Arms (page 83)
- Relaxation Position (page 48): Chin Tucks and Neck Rolls (page 52)
- Bridge with Band (page 159)
- Hip Rolls with Ribcage Closure (page 103)
- Single Leg Stretch (page 121)
- Diamond Leg Lowers (page 128)
- Side Kick Series: Small Circles (page 141)
- Diamond Press Salute with Leg Lift (page 107)
- Box Push Ups (page 150)
- Rest Position with Deep Abdominal Breathing (page 108)
- Pelvic Roll Backs with Leg Slide (page 131)
- High Kneeling Lunge Side Reach (page 105)
- Standing Back Bend with Arm Circles (page 185)

WORKOUT 7

- Ribcage Closure with Wall Slide and Heel Raises (page 81)
- High Kneeling Lunge Waist Twists (page 98)
- Relaxation Position (page 48): Chin Tucks and Neck Rolls (page 52)
- Spine Curls with Ribcage Closure (page 91)
- Curl Ups with Double Knee Fold (page 93)
- Double Leg Stretch Prep (page 122)
- The Hundred (page 124)
- Side-lying Knee Cross Overs (page 89)
- Dart with Side Reach and Floating Arm (page 183)
- One-armed Cat (page 96)
- Rest Position (page 108)
- Back Bridge (page 162)
- Dynamic Lunges with Biceps Curls (page 173)
- Roll Downs with Weights (page 112)

WORKOUT 8

- Seated Long Frog Side Reach (page 53)
- Seated Scarf Breathing (page 62)
- Relaxation Position (page 48):
  Chin Tucks and Neck Rolls (page 52)
- Knee Rolls with Ribcage Closure (page 73)
- Basic Bridge (page 158)
- Oblique Curl Ups with Further Reach (page 117)
- Diamond Leg Lowers (page 128)
- Butterflies (page 101)
- Lizard (page 178)
- Table Top with Flies (page 145)
- Rest Position (page 108)
- Pelvic Roll Backs with Leg Slide (page 131)
- Pilates Squats with Band (page 169)

WORKOUT 9

- Pilates Stance (page 60): Heel Raises and Single
  Floating Arms (page 83)
- High Kneeling Waist Twist (page 97)
- Relaxation Position (page 48):
  Chin Tucks and Neck Rolls (page 52)
- Spine Curls with Knee Opening (page 91)
- Curl Ups with Double Knee Fold (page 93)
- Double Leg Stretch Prep (page 122)
- The Hundred – your level (page 124)
- Side Twist Prep (page 138)
- Diamond Press Salute with Leg Lift (page 107)
- Box Push Ups (page 150)
- Rest Position with Deep Abdominal Breathing
  (page 108)
- Back Bridge and Knee Fold (page 163)
- Roll Downs with Weights (page 112)

WORKOUT 10

- Relaxation Position (page 48):
  Chin Tucks and Neck Rolls (page 52)
- The Hundred Breathing Pattern (page 63)
- Knee Rolls with Ribcage Closure (page 73)
- Spine Curls with Arm Circles (page 91)
- Oblique Curl Ups with Further Reach (page 117)
- Single Leg Stretch (page 121)
- Diamond Leg Lowers (page 128)
- Arm Openings with Weights (page 101)
- Dart with Two Floating Arms (page 181)
- One-armed Cat (page 96)
- Rest Position (page 108)
- High Kneeling Lunge Side Reach (page 105)
- Dynamic Lunges with Bicep Curls (page 173)
- Pilates Squats with Band (page 169)

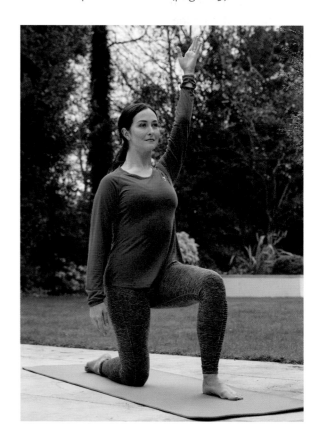

Medium workouts level 1–6
(25–30 MINUTES)

We've given you seven workouts here to try in rotation. Remember that you can add extra exercises for problem areas into the middle of these workouts.

WORKOUT 1
- Pilates Stance Heel Raises with Arm Circles (page 84)
- Standing Side Reach (page 104)
- Relaxation Position (page 48): Chin Tucks and Neck Rolls (page 52)
- Shoulder Drops with Weights (page 78)
- Knee Rolls with Ribcage Closure (page 73)
- Curl Ups with Knee Opening (page 93)
- Spine Curls with Knee Fold (page 91)
- Oblique Curl Ups with Further Reach (page 117)
- Single Leg Stretch Toe Taps (page 120)
- Arm Openings with Weights (page 101)
- Oyster with Band (page 88)
- Torpedo with Hamstring Curls (page 143)
- Diamond Press Salute with Leg Lift (page 107)
- Cobra Prep (page 174) or Full Cobra (page 176)
- Table Top with Flies (page 145)
- One-armed Cat (page 96)
- Rest Position with Deep Abdominal Breathing (page 108)
- Pelvic Roll Backs with Bicep Curls (page 134)
- Pretzel Back Bridge (page 164)
- High Kneeling Lunge Waist Twist (page 98)
- Dynamic Lunges with Double Floating Arms (page 172)
- Roll Downs and Heel Raise (page 112)

WORKOUT 2
- Ribcage Closure with Wall Slide and Heel Raises (page 81)
- Standing Waist Twist (page 97)
- The Leg Shaper (page 156)
- Relaxation Position (page 48): Chin Tucks and Neck Rolls (page 52)
- Bridge with Band (page 159)
- Hip Rolls with Ribcage Closure (page 103)
- Curls Ups with Leg Slide (page 93)
- Double Leg Stretch (page 123)
- Diamond Leg Lowers (page 128)
- The Hundred Breathing Pattern (page 63)
- Side-lying Knee Cross Overs (page 89)
- Butterflies (page 101)
- Cobra Prep (page 174) or Full Cobra (page 176)
- Lizard (page 178)
- Table Top with Arm Salute and Knee Bend (page 77)
- Rest Position (page 108)
- Arm Weights Sequence: Bicep Curls, Chest Presses, Backstroke Arms, Flies (page 151)
- Dynamic Side Twist Prep (page 139)
- High Kneeling Lunge Side Reach (page 105)
- Dynamic Lunges with Double Floating Arms (page 172)
- Roll Downs with Weights and Heel Raises (page 113)

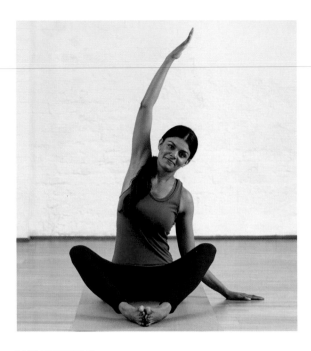

WORKOUT 3

WORKOUT 4

WORKOUT 5

- Pilates Stance with Double Floating Arms (page 83)
- Standing Side Reach (page 104)
- Pilates Squats with Band (page 169)
- High Kneeling Waist Twists (page 97)
- Relaxation position (page 48):
  Chin Tucks and Neck Rolls (page 52)
- Knee Rolls with Ribcage Closure (page 73)
- Bridge with Band (page 159)
- Curl Ups with Leg Slide (page 93)
- Oblique Curl Ups with Further Reach (page 117)
- Double Leg Stretch (page 123)
- The Hundred (page 124)
- Oyster with Band (page 88)
- Side-lying Knee Cross Overs (page 89)
- Arm Openings with Weights (page 101)
- Cobra Prep (page 174) or Full Cobra (page 176)
- Half Star (page 86)
- Table Top with Salute and Knee Bends (page 77)
- Rest Position (page 108)
- Pelvic Roll Backs with Knee Fold (page 132)
- Back Bridge, Knee Fold, Extend, and Lower (page 164)
- The Leg Shaper (page 156)
- Dynamic Lunges with Biceps Curls (page 173)
- Roll Downs and Heel Raise (page 112)

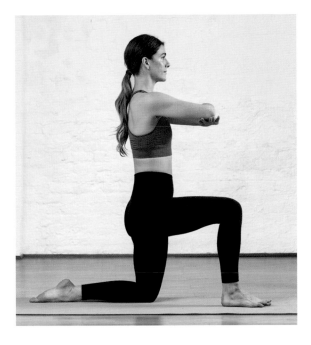

WORKOUT 6

- Relaxation Position (page 48):
  Chin Tucks and Neck Rolls (page 52)
- Shoulder Drops (page 78)
- The Hundred Breathing Pattern (page 63)
- Knee Rolls with Ribcage Closure (page 73)
- Spine Curls with Knee Opening (page 91)
- Hip Rolls with Ribcage Closure (page 103)
- Curl Ups with Leg Slide (page 93)
- Double Leg Stretch (page 123)
- Diamond Leg Lowers (page 128)
- Arm Openings with Weights (page 101)
- Side Kick Series: Small Circles (page 141)
- Diamond Press Salute with Leg Lift (page 107)
- Lizard (page 178)
- Prone Beats (page 177)
- One Arm Box Push Ups (page 150)
- Cat (page 95)
- Rest Position (page 108)
- Back Bridge and Knee Fold (page 163)
- Pelvic Roll Backs with Rowing Variation (page 136)
- Standing Side Reach (page 104)
- Waist Twist in a Not So Static Standing Lunge (page 99)
- Roll Downs (page 110)

WORKOUT 7

- Seated Long Frog with Side Reach (page 53)
- Relaxation Position (page 48):
  Chin Tucks and Neck Rolls (page 52)
- Deep Abdominal Breathing (page 63)
- Arm Circles (page 84)
- Knee Openings, Arms Up (page 69)
- Spine Curls with Knee Fold (page 91)
- Hip Rolls with Leg Extension (page 103)
- Curl Ups with Double Knee Fold (page 93)
- Single Leg Stretch (page 121)
- The Hundred – your level (page 124)
- Torpedo with Extra Leg Lift (page 143)
- Butterflies (page 101)
- Diamond Press Salute with Leg Lifts (page 107)
- Dart with Side Reach (page 182)
- Cat (page 95)
- Dynamic Side Twist Prep (page 139)
- Pelvic Roll Backs with Leg Slide (page 131)
- Pretzel Back Bridge (page 164)
- High Kneeling Lunge with Waist Twists (page 98)
- Standing Hand Weights Sequence: Biceps Press, Chest Expansion (page 153)
- Dynamic Lunges with Double Floating Arms (page 172)
- Pilates Squats with Heel Raise (page 169)

Longer workouts level 1–6
(45–50 MINUTES)

This is the ultimate treat for me... a full Pilates session. Mind and body working together to savour the joy of movement. Beats chocolate every time! (As before, add some Deep Abdominal Breathing (page 63) whenever you feel the need for release.)

WORKOUT 1

- Pilates Squats with Double Floating Arms (page 153)
- Standing Side Reach (page 104)
- High Kneeling Lunge Waist Twists (page 98)
- Seated Scarf Breathing (page 62)
- Relaxation Position (page 48):
  Chin Tucks and Neck Rolls (page 52)
- Shoulder Drops (page 78)
- Arm Circles (page 84)
- Bridge and Knee Fold (page 159)
- Hip Rolls with Leg Extension (page 103)
- Curl Ups with Double Knee Fold (page 93)
- Oblique Curl Ups with Further Reach (page 117)
- Double Leg Stretch (page 123)
- Criss Cross (page 118)
- Butterflies (page 101)
- Side-lying Knee Cross Overs (page 89)
- Arm Weights Sequence: Bicep Curls, Chest Presses, Backstroke Arms, Flies (page 151)
- Dart with Side Reach (page 182)
- Lizard (page 178)
- Table Top with Arm Salute and Knee Bends (page 77)
- Cat (page 95)
- Pelvic Roll Backs with Rowing Prep (page 135)
- Pretzel Back Bridge (page 164)
- Dynamic Lunges with Double Floating Arms (page 172)
- Standing Back Bend with Arm Circles (page 185)
- Roll Downs with Weights (page 112)

WORKOUT 2

- Ribcage Closure with Wall Slides (page 81)
- Standing Side Reach (page 104)
- The Leg Shaper (page 156)
- Relaxation Position (page 48):
  Chin Tucks and Neck Rolls (page 52)
- Shoulder Drops (page 78)
- Double Knee Fold with Arms Up (page 70)
- Spine Curls with Arm Circles (page 91)
- Curl Ups with Leg Slide (page 93)
- Single Leg Stretch (page 121)
- The Hundred – your level (page 124)
- Diamond Leg Lowers (page 128)
- Oyster with Band (page 88)
- Side Kick Series: Small Circles (page 141)
- Arm Openings with Weights (page 101)
- Cobra Prep (page 174) or Full Cobra (page 176)
- Half Star (page 86)
- Prone Beats (page 177)
- One-armed Cat (page 96)
- Rest Position (page 108)
- Dynamic Side Twist Prep (page 139)
- Leg Pull Back (page 167)
- Pelvic Roll Backs with Knee Fold (page 132)
- High Kneeling Lunge Side Reach (page 105)
- Dynamic Lunges with Double Floating Arms
  (page 172)
- Pilates Squats with Bicep Curls (page 169)
- Roll Downs (page 110)

WORKOUT 3

- Relaxation Position (page 48):
  Chin Tucks and Neck Rolls (page 52)
- Shoulder Drops (page 78)
- Knee Rolls with Ribcage Closure (page 73)
- Basic Bridge (page 158)
- Curl Ups with Double Knee Fold (page 93)
- Hip Rolls with Leg Extension (page 103)
- Criss Cross (page 118)
- The Hundred – your level (page 124)
- Diamond Leg Lowers (page 128)
- Oyster with Band (page 88)
- Torpedo with Extra Leg Lift (page 143)
- Butterflies (page 101)
- Dart with Two Floating Arms (page 181)
- Lizard with Legs (page 179)
- One-armed Cat (page 96)
- Table Top with Flies and Lifted Leg (page 145)
- Rest Position (page 108)
- Pelvic Roll Backs, Rowing Prep with Rotation
  (page 136)
- Back Bridge, Knee Fold, Extend, and Lower
  (page 164)
- High Kneeling Lunge Side Reach (page 105)
- Standing Hand Weights Sequence: Biceps Press,
  Chest Expansion (page 153)
- Dynamic Lunges with Single Floating Arm
  (alternate)(page 172)
- Standing Back Bend with Arm Circles (page 185)

WORKOUT 4

- Seated Long Frog Side Reach (page 53)
- Seated Scarf Breathing (page 62)
- Relaxation Position (page 48):
  Chin Tucks and Neck Rolls (page 52)
- Arm Circles (page 84)
- Spine Curls with Knee Opening (page 91)
- Hip Rolls with Ribcage Closure (page 103)
- Curl Ups with Leg Slide (page 93)
- Oblique Curl Ups with Further Reach (page 117)
- Single Leg Stretch (page 121)
- Double Leg Stretch (page 123)
- Side-lying Knee Cross Overs (page 89)
- Arm Openings with Weights (page 101)
- Diamond Press Salute (page 107)
- Cobra Prep (page 174) or Full Cobra (page 176)
- Prone Beats (page 177)
- Cat (page 95)
- Leg Pull Front (page 148) or Table Top with
  Knee Bend (page 77)
- Rest Position (page 108)
- Pelvic Roll Backs with Single or Double
  Leg Slide (pages 131–132)
- Pretzel Back Bridge (page 164)
- Waist Twist in High Kneeling Lunge (page 98)
- Dynamic Lunges with Bicep Curls (page 173)
- Roll Downs with Weights and Double Floating
  Arms and Heel Raises (page 113)

WORKOUT 5

- Pilates Stance with Heel Raises (page 60)
- Standing Side Reach (page 104)
- The Leg Shaper (page 156)
- Relaxation Position (page 48):
  Chin Tucks and Neck Rolls (page 52)
- Knee Rolls with Ribcage Closure (page 73)
- Basic Bridge (page 158)
- Hip Rolls with Leg Extension (page 103)
- Curl Ups with Double Knee Fold (page 93)
- Oblique Curl Ups with Further Reach (page 117)
- The Hundred – your level (page 124)
- Criss Cross (page 118)
- Torpedo with Extra Leg Lift (page 143)
- Butterflies (page 101)
- Arm Weights Sequence: Bicep Curls,
  Chest Presses, Backstroke Arms, Flies (page 151)
- Lizard with Legs (page 179)
- Cobra Prep (page 174) or Full Cobra (page 176)
- Prone Beats (page 177)
- Cat (page 95)
- Rest Position (page 108)
- One Arm Box Push Ups (page 150)
- Back Bridge and Knee Fold (page 163)
- Pelvic Roll Backs with Rowing Prep (page 135)
- High Kneeling Lunge Side Reach (page 105)
- Dynamic Lunges with Bicep Curls (page 173)
- Roll Downs (page 110)

A healthy future

By the time you reach this page you should be well on your way to being fitter, healthier and in your best shape ever. Small changes to your lifestyle have become as routine as daily brushing your teeth. You are feeling as good as you look. Congratulations!

But it is not just your life you've changed; you have set an example for generations to come. This is so important, especially with the current worrying rise in obesity levels in children. If this trend continues, the next generation may be struggling with significant health problems. Children follow our lead. If ever you need extra motivation to maintain this healthy way of life bear in mind that a mother's lifestyle and activity levels can have a huge impact on their children's health.

A Norwegian study published in 2018 discovered that if a mother lost or gained weight, her children did too. The conclusion was if parents adopt behaviours that lead to obesity, these behaviours are mirrored by their children.

We opened this book by saying that we all have a responsibility not only to ourselves, but to our families and children to live a healthy life. I cannot think of a better gift to give my children and grandchildren – the gift of a healthy future.

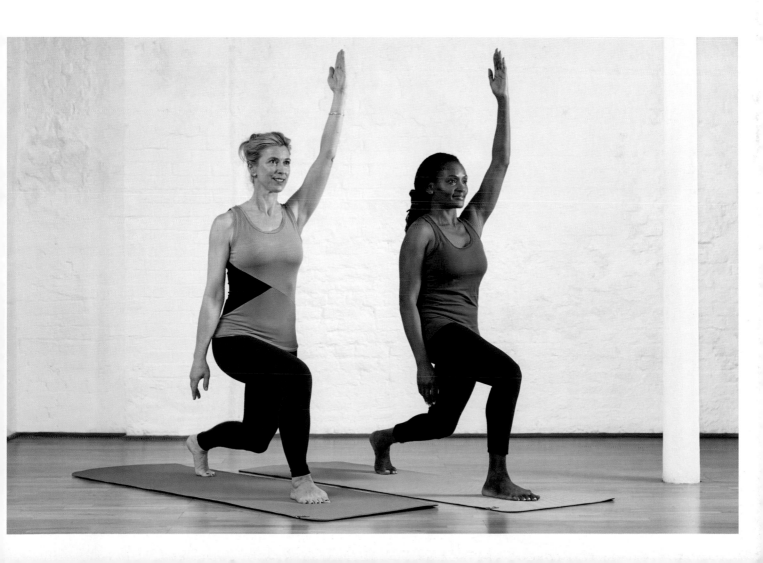

Resources

BODY CONTROL PILATES

For more information on Body Control Pilates, local teachers, classes, teacher training courses, books, equipment and DVDs: www.bodycontrolpilates.com

If you enjoy the exercises and workouts in this book, you will love our online video subscription channel with Shape Up workouts presented by Lynne and Sarah, masterclasses, tutorials and lots more for public and teachers alike: www.bodycontrolpilatescentral. vhx.tv

Our Body Control Pilates flagship studio and headquarters are based in Bloomsbury, central London. Visit us and the Rosetta Stone at The British Museum all in one trip!

The Body Control Pilates Centre
35 Little Russell Street
London WC1A 2HH
Email: info@bodycontrol.co.uk
Tel: +44 (0)20 7636 8900
Facebook: www.facebook.com/
BodyControlPilates
Instagram @bodycontrolpilates and
@bcpcentral
Twitter @bodycontrol

CARDIOVASCULAR HEALTH

For heart health information:
www.bhf.org.uk
www.heart.org

For advice on how to prevent injury while exercising aerobically:
www.heart.org/en/healthy-living/fitness/fitness-basics/preventing-injury-during-your-workout

If you are looking for an aerobics instructor or a personal trainer, make sure that they have an externally accredited qualification that meets the relevant national standards.

NUTRITION

For nutrition information:
www.nutrition.org.uk

Helen Ford is Head of Nutrition at Glenville Nutrition Clinic:
www.glenvillenutrition.com
Email: reception@glenvillenutrition.com
Tel: + 44 (0) 1892 515905
Instagram @helenfordnutrition

OBESITY AND EATING DISORDERS

For information about obesity:
www.britishobesitysociety.org
www.nhs.uk/conditions/obesity
www.obesity.org

For information on eating disorders:
www.beateatingdisorders.org.uk
www.nationaleatingdisorders.org
www.nhs.uk/conditions/eating-disorders

STRESS

If stress is becoming overwhelming, speak to your doctor.

For stress management:
www.stress.org.uk

For information on Forest Schools:
www.forestschoolassociation.org

If you are interested in meditation:
www.britishmeditationsociety.com
To help you meditate we highly recommend *Mindfulness Meditations*, guided meditation tracks by Dr Mark Williams from Oxford Meditation Centre:
https://mbct.co.uk/cd-set/

SLEEP

If you have trouble sleeping and feel it is affecting your health, speak to your doctor.

For insomnia advice:
www.nhs.uk/conditions/insomnia

Index

An Hachette UK Company
www.hachette.co.uk

First published in Great Britain in 2020 by
Kyle Books, an imprint of Kyle Cathie Ltd
Carmelite House
50 Victoria Embankment
London EC4Y 0DZ
www.kylebooks.co.uk

ISBN: 978 0 85783 589 5

Text copyright 2020 © Lynne Robinson
Design and layout copyright 2020 © Kyle Books

Distributed in the US by Hachette Book Group,
1290 Avenue of the Americas,
4th and 5th Floors, New York, NY 10104

Distributed in Canada by Canadian Manda Group,
664 Annette St., Toronto, Ontario, Canada M6S 2C8

Lynne Robinson is hereby identified as the author
of this work in accordance with Section 77 of the
Copyright, Designs and Patents Act 1988.

Publisher Joanna Copestick
Editorial director Judith Hannam
Editor Vicky Orchard
Editorial assistant Sarah Kyle
Design Ketchup
Photography Claire Pepper
Production Lucy Carter

A Cataloguing in Publication record for this title
is available from the British Library

Printed and bound in China

10 9 8 7 6 5 4 3 2 1

LYNNE'S ACKNOWLEDGEMENTS

I celebrated my 65th birthday whilst writing this book. I've been teaching Pilates now for 25 years and I can confidently say that I'm in better shape now, fitter and more flexible, than I was when I was 40! But it's not just my body that Pilates has shaped, it's my life. What a journey and what wonderful people I've met along the way. All my dear clients, our talented tutors at our teacher training centre, our incredible growing Body Control teaching community. This book is the culmination of all their work and I'm deeply grateful for their loyalty and dedication.

But, in particular, I want to thank my dearest friend and fellow tutor Sarah Clennell, who agreed, after a few glasses of bubbly, to help me with the book. Sarah's endless creativity is equally matched by her technical expertise. We had so much fun as we, quite literally, rolled around the floor, inventing new and adapting old exercises. I owe her so much; words are inadequate to express my gratitude on both a professional and personal level.

Then there's Helen, our incredibly talented and highly qualified nutritionist. It's rare to someone so wise who is also so lovely! You have been unbelievably generous with your knowledge. Your chapter may be short, but it's packed with life-changing advice.

And then there's all the other people without whom this book would never have been published. From the point of signing, with the help of our agent Michael Alcock, our commissioning editor Judith Hannam, to the amazing designer Megan Smith. And, at the helm, the beautiful, calm, encouraging and patient hand of Vicky Orchard our editor. (Vicky has the rare and remarkable skill of being able to decipher my handwriting. No mean feat, believe me.)

As for Claire Pepper, our photographer and her team of lovely assistants, I can only say I was blown away by her calm professionalism and creative genius. Nothing phased her, no request too much trouble, no angle impossible! I've never laughed so much on a photoshoot!

Our stunning models: Heidi, Rachel, Harriet, Zoe, Tunde, Ulrike, Ai Lin, Jonelle, I'm sure you'll agree they are fabulous. Thank you so much for agreeing to be part of this project. I hope you all enjoyed it as much as we did.

Then to make us all look the part we can thank the make-up team – Katrin Rees, Emma Kingsman and Natasha Sheridan. My hair stylist, Dene Graham at Martyn Maxey, has been with me since I took up Pilates. Dene you are never allowed to retire. If you do, I'll have to fly over to Italy to see you! I also want to thank the always bubbly staff at The Gallery, Southborough, Tunbridge Wells – my visits are amongst the highlights of my week!

Alice Asquith, thank you for letting us use your fabulous bamboo clothing...so comfortable and so flattering. Perfect for Pilates.

And finally, I need to thank my wonderful family. We've had a tough year, challenge after challenge. Well, together we've faced them and emerged stronger and closer. Pilates might have given me the physical and emotional strength to cope, but you all are, and will always be, my true inspiration.

SARAH'S ACKNOWLEDGEMENTS

A huge thank you to Lynne Robinson for putting her trust in me to help with the book. Lynne has always been a steady support over many years. She is an inspiring role model whom I very much respect and admire. We had fun creating ideas together with ease and flow. Most of all, I cherish her friendship.

Thanks to the entire Robinson family for supporting me. Giving me opportunities to grow and develop with interesting challenges and adventures over the years.

It's been a pleasure working with the entire team involved in the creative process to bring the book together. What awesome talent!

HELEN'S ACKNOWLEDGEMENTS

I would firstly like to thank Lynne for giving me the opportunity to contribute to this wonderful book. She is a remarkable lady with passion and a kind heart and soul.

Thank you to my beautiful family for giving me the time and headspace to write my chapter. My husband Mike has been so supportive and a constant source of encouragement. To my two beautiful children, Poppy and Jake, for their constant humour and cuddles.

Finally, a big thanks to the photography team for making me look "the part"!